About the Authors

CHRISTOPHER KENNEDY LAWFORD holds a bachelor of arts degree from Tufts University, a Juris Doctor from Boston College Law School, and a master's certification in clinical psychology from Harvard Medical School. He has worked extensively in Hollywood as an actor, lawyer, executive, and producer, and his first book, *Symptoms of Withdrawal*, debuted on the *New York Times* bestseller list. He is also the editor of *Moments of Clarity: Voices from the Front Lines of Addiction and Recovery*. He lives in Marina del Rey, California.

DIANA SYLVESTRE, MD, is a physician-researcher and faculty member in the Department of Medicine at the University of California, San Francisco. She received her education at Harvard Medical School and trained in internal medicine at Brigham and Women's Hospital, a teaching affiliate of Harvard, and is a specialist in addiction medicine. In 1998 she founded O.A.S.I.S.—Organization to Achieve Solutions in Substance-Abuse—a nonprofit community-based medical clinic that provides education and treatment services to underserved patients with hepatitis C, and continues to serve as its executive director. Dr. Sylvestre is the president of the California Hepatitis Alliance, a statewide advocacy organization formed to develop and advance sound viral hepatitis public policy, and is active in many other hepatitis advocacy organizations.

Healing Hepatitis C

**A PATIENT AND A DOCTOR ON
THE EPIDEMIC'S FRONT LINES TELL YOU HOW TO**

- Recognize When You Are at Risk
- Understand Hepatitis C Tests
- Talk to Your Doctor About Hepatitis C
- Advocate for Yourself and Others

Christopher Kennedy Lawford
and Diana Sylvestre, MD

HARPER

NEW YORK • LONDON • TORONTO • SYDNEY

HARPER

HEALING HEPATITIS C. Copyright © 2009 by Christopher Kennedy Lawford and Diana Sylvestre. All rights reserved. Printed in the United States of America. No part of this book may be used or reproduced in any manner whatsoever without written permission except in the case of brief quotations embodied in critical articles and reviews. For information address Harper-Collins Publishers, 10 East 53rd Street, New York, NY 10022.

HarperCollins books may be purchased for educational, business, or sales promotional use. For information please write: Special Markets Department, HarperCollins Publishers, 10 East 53rd Street, New York, NY 10022.

FIRST EDITION

Designed by Joy O'Meara

Library of Congress Cataloging-in-Publication Data is available upon request.

ISBN 978-0-06-178368-5

09 10 11 12 13   OV/RRD   10 9 8 7 6 5 4 3 2

To the many whose struggles inspired us

Contents

Preface

H epatitis C? What's that?"
    "How did I get it?"
"What about my family and friends?"
"Is there a treatment?"
"Am I going to die?"

These are just a few of the many good questions we hear all the time: one of us as a patient and the other as a doctor, both of us hepatitis C educators and advocates. Even though more than four million persons in the United States and nearly two hundred million people worldwide are affected by hepatitis C, it is still hard to get straightforward answers. We hope to change that here.

Our own paths first converged through our common interests in hepatitis C activism and the conviction that strong advocacy leads to good health policy. We both serve in leadership positions in the California Hepatitis Alliance (CalHEP), a statewide organization that seeks to improve California's legislative approach to the viral hepatitis epidemic, and we continue to meet with our governor and other policy makers on an ongoing basis to educate them about this condition and to inform sound public health policies in our state.

Despite our vastly different backgrounds, we came to recognize that our personal journeys in hepatitis C had significant parallels. Neither of us set out to be an expert on hepatitis C or to advocate for awareness and treatment: Hepatitis C had been an imposed struggle rather than a visionary process. For both of us our initial ignorance and frustration was ultimately supplanted by growth, hope, and success. And to be honest we have both been well served by our tendencies toward hardheadedness.

This is a different kind of hepatitis C book. It takes the form of a conversation between us, as we speak and respond to each other about our shared experiences, struggles, and successes with hepatitis C. But although we speak to each other, we are really speaking to you. You will come to learn about hepatitis C much as we did: in a gradual way, from trial and effort, from ourselves as well as the other patients whose struggles are recounted here.

Having hepatitis C can be a transformative, "forty days and forty nights" kind of experience. It is tough. But in these personal stories of confronting stigma and misinformation, fears and frustrations, you will find a sourcebook for medical and treatment information: what hepatitis C is and what it does, what to expect during treatment, how to communicate with your physician, ways to find the support you need, and how to advocate for yourself, your friends, and loved ones. But most of all we hope to walk you through the process of facing the diagnosis and treatment head-on, to show you that it is possible to get through this hepatitis C thing—and to be cured—without surrendering your life to it.

Christopher Kennedy Lawford
Diana Sylvestre, MD

Healing Hepatitis C

Chapter 1

Exposures

I want to test you for hepatitis C and HIV." That was what the guy in the white coat, Dr. Rob Huizenga, told me after he finished my workup. It was 2000, he was my new internist, and I'd walked into his office to deal with a sty in my right eye. I'd just returned from shooting the movie *Thirteen Days* in the jungles of the Philippines, and I wanted to make sure I hadn't picked up some weird eye-eating disease. I figured that while I was there it might be a good time to get a routine physical. It was my first visit, but I felt a connection to him almost immediately. Dr. Huizenga is one of the top internists in Los Angeles, and he happens to be one of those big, blond, perfect physical specimens—as if Rutger Hauer had moved to LA and gone to medical school instead of starring in *Blade Runner*. His hobby is sports medicine, and he was the Los Angeles Raiders' team doctor for their entire tenure in LA before they moved back to Oakland where they belonged.

He's generally a no-nonsense-type guy. I liked him and I trusted him. That turned out to be very important to me over the next eighteen months.

I knew why he wanted to run those tests. I'd been in recovery for fifteen years, but I'd been a serious drug and alcohol user for the fifteen years before that. I used needles. And syringes, cottons, cookers, rinse water, whatever it took, and I shared with other drug addicts. It was a necessary thing to do. And in those years we didn't know anything about long-term, chronic, serious diseases. You could catch something really unpleasant but probably not fatal, like hepatitis B, and you might even die from endocarditis, which is an infection of the heart lining. My cousin David suffered from that for years before the disease of addiction finally killed him. But I didn't know anything about the real dangers of the risky behavior I was engaged in until after I'd stopped using drugs and alcohol.

I got clean and sober just before HIV really started spreading. Hepatitis C? That wasn't on anyone's radar. Oh, I knew about hepatitis. I'm the poster boy for hepatitis. I'd gotten hepatitis B in my early twenties from a dirty needle, and I'd spent a very bad week at my grandmother's house in Palm Beach, thinking I might die and just wanting to get better so I could get back to doing what I'd been doing. And then, five years after I cleaned up, I was at a lunchtime recovery meeting in Santa Monica, eating a perfectly delicious tuna salad, when I was introduced to that nasty virus known as hepatitis A. I didn't know it at the time but hep A is spread mainly through bad hygiene. For instance, infected food-prep workers who don't wash their hands after using the bathroom can spread tiny amounts of virus-loaded fecal matter onto a piece of lettuce, turning a harmless tuna salad into a bioweapon. Now enjoy your lunch!

After I had been sober for five years I began to hear about an addition to the hepatitis alphabet—hep C. A few of the folks trudging alongside me on the recovery road of happy destiny were getting diagnosed with hepatitis C, and it didn't sound good. The whispers I heard in the meetings were that this new disease could chew up your liver and put you in line for a transplant—maybe even kill you. There was a treatment, but nobody was speaking very enthusiastically about it. Then two friends of mine I'd run with back in the day were diagnosed with hep C. That's when I got scared. If my mates had it, maybe I did too. One of them began treatment. This was in the early days, when treatment consisted of injecting a drug called interferon into one's thigh daily or several times a week. After six months or so of being depressed and feeling as if he had the flu, he was told by his doctor that the treatment hadn't worked.

The impression I got from his experience was that the treatment was worse than the disease, which scared me to death and convinced me that I should never get tested. But whenever I ran into one of these guys my fear would spike, and I'd have the conversation with myself. Whenever I get scared I start talking to myself. Well, no—that's not quite accurate. What happens is, the voices in my head start talking to each other and I just go along for a terrifying ride. The voices would have a field day during my eleven months of treatment for hepatitis C. They'd make stupid jokes to ward off fear, and they were often pretty ignorant about medical procedures, including liver transplants. And one of them was really, *really* against the whole idea of treatment.

JUNKIE CHRIS:

Why should we get tested? I don't want to shoot some nasty drug into my leg every day that makes me feel like shit, and probably won't work anyway!

SOBER CHRIS:

We should get tested. This thing can kill!

JUNKIE CHRIS:

Come on. We look good, we feel good, we're not sick. We dodged another bullet, man.

SOBER CHRIS:

But what if we have it?

JUNKIE CHRIS:

We'll be spending lots of time at the zoo, checking out which baboon we'll be getting a liver from. . . .

Eventually the sober, more prudent Chris prevailed, and I started to think seriously about getting tested. A friend from college had become an emergency-room doctor, and

I asked him to test me for hep C. I didn't want to go to a doctor I didn't know and have to explain why I thought I needed the test. There was a certain amount of shame and fear in me at the time, even though I had dealt openly with my addiction—but this was a serious, potentially fatal disease. A disease I didn't fully understand. Was I contagious? Would I become some sort of pariah? Was I looking at dragging around a swollen belly as my liver slowly shut down and I turned yellower and yellower? Shit! This was not good. It felt like my past was catching up to me, after so many years of sobriety. Was this some kind of punishment for my misspent youth? Finally my doctor friend gave me a blood workup and a week or so later said, "You're fine. You don't have it." What a relief. Junkie Chris was right—another bullet dodged.

After that hepatitis C was totally off the table for me. I did worry about HIV, but if I was afraid of getting tested for hepatitis C, I was terrified of getting an HIV test. I was pretty sure I was safe, because the last time I remembered putting a needle in my arm was in 1981, just as the first cases of what would become AIDS were being identified in the United States. But let's be clear— a drug addict's memory is anything *but* clear, and there was always a fear that I'd gotten sober only to die of AIDS years later. It seemed like the perfect ironic twist, an exclamation point on a privileged life gone unappreciated and unrealized.

So here's what I told Dr. Huizenga ten years after my emergency-room test for hep C. "I haven't had an HIV test and I probably should have one, but don't bother with the hepatitis C test because I've already been tested for that, and I don't have it."

Fortunately for me I was standing in front of a doctor who wasn't going to let me weasel out of what I needed to do. We'd just gone over my history, and he was not going to take no for an answer. He said, "Look, your liver function tests are a little high but in the normal range. Not high enough to dictate a test, but given your history I think it's a good idea."

"Yeah, my LFTs have always been a little high. That's normal for me. They've been that way for years." That was another reason I knew my liver was fine. While I was drinking and using drugs, doctors warned me that I had elevated liver function tests. I always assumed that was a result of my substance abuse, and sure enough, when I got sober, the liver function levels dropped down to normal. High normal but normal.

"Okay," he said. "But humor me. I want to see for myself."

I did a couple of things right. I picked a doctor who could handle the truth about my history, and then I told him the truth. I'm sure that influenced his insistence on testing, and that in turn might have saved my life. Rob told me later that if he'd been testing only patients with high liver functions out of the normal range, I wouldn't have qualified.

I got blood taken for the tests, and then I more or less forgot that somewhere deep in the basement of some building, in a blood lab on the Westside of Los Angeles, a lab technician was testing my blood, looking for the presence of not one but two life-threatening illnesses. After all, I was pretty sure I didn't have HIV, and I *knew* I didn't have hepatitis C.

Two weeks later I got a call from Dr. Huizenga. "I've got good news and I've got bad news." Let's get something straight: A doctor calling up and saying he's got good news and bad news is never good news.

You can always count on an addict to go for immediate gratification before dealing with any unpleasantness.

"What's the good news?" I asked.

"Well, you don't have HIV," Dr. Huizenga responded.

"That's great." I said. "What's the bad news?"

"You *do* have hepatitis C."

"No fucking way!"

Chris isn't the only one to have gotten hepatitis C wrong at first: So did I. And that is something you should understand right up front. You see, I am not a hepatitis C doctor, I am a doctor who treats hepatitis C. That distinction may sound meaningless, but for me it has been central to everything I have done in this field. It means this: I am not a trained hepatologist; I don't belong to "the club." I am a specialist in addiction medicine. I didn't start out with a burning desire to follow the traditional training path and take on the hepatitis C virus. I came to understand hepatitis C much as you probably have: I had no choice in the matter.

The kinds of hepatitis C patients I like to care for are rejected by society and the traditional medical system. They are poor, uninsured, mentally ill, and homeless. Many have decades-long histories of drug use before they surface in my clinic. But inside those patients is the fundamental kind of warmth and gratitude and honesty that many people never see, because it is a challenge to bring them out. And so I eventually came to treat large numbers of hepatitis C patients like these for no good reason other than I had to: There was no other option at the time. No one else would do it. If you don't want to read about this kind of hepatitis C patient, now would be the time to stop.

In my case the story starts in 1995. I had just taken a new job doing medical intakes at a drug treatment program in San Leandro, California. Dr. Carolyn Schuman was the medical director, and she ran the good kind of community-based nonprofit treatment program that cared about its patients. At the time I didn't know all that much about taking care of drug users. I thought it would be something challenging and interesting to learn.

Unfortunately, like many drug programs for poor people, the facility was dingy and depressing. The floor was cracking in half where the doublewide building had originally been joined. The walls wore years of scuffs and scratches, and windows were crusted with dust and cobwebs. Doors didn't quite fit and sometimes locked themselves shut. The bathroom reeked like the ones in a bus station; it hardly improved when a gallon of disinfectant, my first donation, was dumped on the floor. I came to understand that when you are poor and you are addicted, you don't complain about these things. No one is going to pretty things up just to get your business. And by the time you enter treatment you figure: This is what I deserve.

My job was to interview new patients, do a physical exam, and check some basic blood tests to make sure all was reasonably well and that starting drug treatment was safe— as if the alternative could ever be considered safer. It was usually a matter of getting through the history and physical as quickly as possible because patients in drug withdrawal are not feeling well, and then reviewing the laboratory tests later as they became available.

But in going through those results, I kept coming across something unusual. What is going on with these liver tests? I wondered. One after another of my new patients had elevated liver enzymes, suggesting some kind of problem but not really pointing in one direction or another. Liver enzyme abnormalities can mean a million things. The ones I was noticing were usually minor and intermittent, and often they had been present for years without attracting attention. Few patients had ever been told that their tests were abnormal, and with far more pressing concerns about stopping drug use, even fewer seemed to care. Was alcohol causing it? Heroin? Cocaine? I had no idea.

I still cringe when I think about that: having no idea that hepatitis C was staring right at me. During my years of fancy education and internal medicine training at Harvard Medical School and Brigham and Women's Hospital in Boston, we would see patients with the strange condition called "non-A, non-B hepatitis" all the time. They had been blood transfusion recipients, hemophiliacs, cardiac surgery patients. We would shrug because there wasn't much to do. For fifteen years we had called it by that strange name because we only knew what it wasn't—not hepatitis A, and not hepatitis B—but despite armies of researchers, we didn't know what it *was*.

And then in 1989 the code was cracked. Elegant work by Dr. Michael Houghton and his colleagues at a biotechnology company called Chiron, and the Centers for Disease Control (CDC) in Atlanta, had led to the cloning of the non-A, non-B hepatitis virus. And finally it was given its real name: hepatitis C. It was a scientific tour de force, because at the time the virus had never been visualized, grown in culture, or immunologically defined. Dr. Houghton and Dr. Harvey Alter from the National Institutes of Health (NIH) were subsequently given the Lasker Award for their achievements in hepatitis C—one of the most respected scientific prizes in the world. It was a big exciting deal, this work. I followed it closely.

Within three years, while I was otherwise occupied as a fellow in molecular immunology at Sloan-Kettering Institute in New York City, this remarkable discovery had led to the development of a highly accurate hepatitis C diagnostic test. In 1992 universal screening of the U.S. blood supply began. Until then hepatitis C had been a fairly common consequence of having a blood transfusion. Despite improvements in the blood collection and screening process—the elimination of paid donors, the initiation of mandatory testing for hepatitis B virus protein in 1972 and, starting in 1987, the rejection of donors whose blood had liver enzyme abnormalities or signs of prior exposure to hepatitis B infection—as many as one in twenty transfusion recipients were still infected. The number of people who had been exposed to non-A, non-B hepatitis, now called hepatitis C, was immense: some four million in the United States alone. This unfortunate fact had distracted most of us, including me, from recognizing its even greater impact on the patients that many of us paid little attention to: injection drug users.

To this day a lot of people automatically associate hepatitis C with drug use, failing to recognize how many people were exposed in other ways. That unfortunate misconception still keeps people from asking for the test. In fact in some of the years before we began mandatory testing of the U.S. blood supply, there were nearly two hundred thousand new cases of hepatitis C annually, many of which were contracted from blood transfusions.

What many people don't know is how the two transmission modalities are interrelated: It was not uncommon to offer jail inmates a sentence reduction for donating a unit of blood. Many had been incarcerated for drug-related offenses, and they were happy to comply with a request for blood if there was something in it for them. Unfortunately, being drug users, many were also infected with hepatitis C. It was an unintentional collision of scientific ignorance and uninformed drug policies focused on incarceration instead of treatment. One of my hepatitis C patients proudly showed me his donation card from prison. He had given two gallons of blood.

But there are other ways to get hepatitis C. Even though sex is a pretty inefficient way of transmitting the virus from person to person, about 15 percent of cases are related to sexual transmission. That adds up to a good number, when you're starting from four million. Sometimes hepatitis C is passed from mother to child at the time of birth, and there are needlestick injuries and the like. And in about 10 percent of cases, we just don't know for sure.

What it comes down to is that in those years before we began testing the blood supply, there were so many new cases of hepatitis C each year that people like me didn't notice its immense impact on drug users, even though I should have. In fact, because hepatitis C is so easily transmitted by even small amounts of blood, over 90 percent of current and former needle users in some localities, including mine, had been exposed. Like many, I just hadn't been paying attention. Addicts? They had pretty much been off my radar. Little did I know that they would eventually teach me everything I needed know about hepatitis C.

D r. Huizenga had seen it all before and this wasn't the first time he'd given a patient bad news. It came with the territory. His bedside manner was steady, unflappable; he was ready to make a plan. I, on the other hand, was reeling.

JUNKIE CHRIS:
Nice, Chris. Leave it to you to survive drug addiction, clean up your life, and then die from a disease you got twenty years ago.

SOBER CHRIS:
I'm not going to die. There's been some kind of mistake.

JUNKIE CHRIS:

*Don't be too sure, my man. You weren't very care-
ful back in your "adventuresome youth." I hear this
hep C is a mofo . . . liver cancer, cirrhosis . . . doesn't
sound like too much fun to me. Remember how yellow and hurting your father was when he died? The
cirrhosis had turned his liver into a piece of corru-
gated cardboard.*

SOBER CHRIS:

*Good thing it was me talking to the doctor, not you.
You would've just lied to him.*

JUNKIE CHRIS:

*Where did being honest get us? We have an incurable
disease, and we're scared shitless!*

I got the voices to shut up so I could talk to Dr. Huizenga.

"How is this possible? I was tested years ago and I
was told I didn't have hep C."

"They got it wrong, Chris, but it might not have been
the doctor's fault. The diagnostics were not as good back
then; they're better now," Dr. Huizenga said.

"But I don't feel sick. I feel fine. I really do." I was trying to convince both him and myself I was okay.

"That's not uncommon. Many people with hep C have
no symptoms, maybe fatigue, but nothing else until the
virus begins to significantly damage your liver. Are you
tired?" he asked.

"I guess," I said.

"How tired are you?" Dr. Huizenga pressed.

"Well, Doc, I'm forty-five years old, I have three kids, I'm an actor, I produce segments on an entertainment-news program, and I'm trying to get my dot-com off the ground—I'm tired. Who isn't tired? I don't know how tired I really am. I'm regular tired, I guess, like everyone. Not hepatitis C tired, though. No way," I said, hoping I was right.

But I could see it right there in my chart: "Lawford, Christopher: Hepatitis C antibody screen: Reactive."

"Maybe someone made a mistake. I mean these labs make mistakes all the time—don't they? What if the earlier tests showing I didn't have hep C were right and this test was wrong? And I even think some other doctor told me at some point that I didn't have hep C. I mean, I couldn't swear to it, but how could *two* doctors have screwed up like this?"

In his calm, no-drama, this-is-the-way-it-is kind of way, Dr. Huizenga explained that the results from the test he had given me were accurate and that I shouldn't blame the doctor or doctors who'd told me I didn't have the virus before. In the years since I'd been tested, the hepatitis C screen had become more accurate, and since the rest of my blood tests were in the normal range, no one had thought to have me retested. A lot of people assume that if they have hepatitis C, there'll be something abnormal in the regular liver enzyme tests, but often this isn't the case. Many people with hepatitis C go to the doctor, don't mention that they have a risk factor, and their regular blood tests are completely normal—even though they have hepatitis C. So they don't have the specific hep C test done, and the virus goes undetected for years, even decades. That's one of the reasons hepatitis C is called the "silent killer."

I think back to that time a lot. About how hard it is to hear that you have hepatitis C, even if you think you are prepared. But as hard as it was, I know today that my honesty probably saved my life. There's still so much shame and misinformation out there about hepatitis C, even though there are upward of four million people in the United States alone who have been exposed—about four or five times more than HIV. And because of this shame and misinformation, most of those people don't even know they have it. I have seen in my recovery from addiction how reaching my hand out in solidarity and service can obliterate that shame, radically altering a person's experience with his or her disease. I have seen it in recovery, and I have seen it with hepatitis C. There's a similar stigma with both, a similar shame in talking about them. Whenever I give a presentation, I often talk about my hepatitis C and the fact that I've been cured. Not that long ago I was at a recovery conference, and afterward a woman came up to me and said, "I can't believe you talked about that!" All I could say was, "Talked about what?" She said, "Hepatitis C. I have it and I don't talk to anybody about it."

That's crazy. There's no shame in having hepatitis C, and getting the diagnosis can save your life. Nowadays a lot of people like me who get the diagnosis are cured with treatment. So who cares how you got it? Whether it was from a blood transfusion or a sexual dalliance or, like me, from using drugs in your youth, the important thing is to get the test.

And it is important to talk about it. I like talking about the things I care about. I like talking about addiction and hepatitis C because I know about them. I want to confront the shame and misinformation, because they affect the way we deal with this disease. Even with four million affected Americans, hepatitis C is an issue that is utterly unaddressed on a political, national, and public policy level. Some states have developed plans for confronting this epidemic, but there is little hope of finding the money to implement those plans—there's no political will, even though the problem is only going to get bigger. The CDC estimates that there are upward of twenty thousand new HCV infections every year, and recent research predicts that by the year 2030, annual death rates from hep C will approach twenty thousand—but because many of those new infections occur in the drug-addicted population, it's difficult to get anyone to pay attention. And look what's happening around the world. Outside the United States, there are nearly two hundred million people exposed to hepatitis C. I sat next to a liver specialist working in Egypt at a dinner in Washington, DC, and he told me that 15 percent of the Egyptian population could have this illness. I've learned so much about this public health crisis and what I've learned has motivated me to spend more of my time trying to get lawmakers, healthcare professionals, and the average American motivated to learn—and do—more about it.

But back then, sitting across from my new doctor who had just given me the diagnosis of hepatitis C, none of this was going through my mind. I was not thinking about stigma, or activism, or policies. I was thinking only that I had just heard I had an illness that might kill me and I had no idea what I was going to do about it.

Wouldn't you think, with more than four million Americans and something like two hundred million people in the world exposed to hepatitis C, that the word would be out? That the stigma would be gone? That getting a hepatitis C diagnosis wouldn't elicit such alarm? That our medical system would be more forcefully attacking this epidemic?

You would, but these things take time: It has been only a couple of decades since hepatitis C was first cloned and identified. Compare that with tuberculosis. Robert Koch isolated the tubercle bacillus in 1883, and the antibiotic streptomycin was first determined to be effective against it in 1944, more than sixty years ago. But tuberculosis is still flourishing. In 2005 the World Health Organization (WHO) estimated that there were more than 14 million cases of tuberculosis worldwide and that it had led to nearly 1.6 million deaths. Similarly, the *Treponema pallidum* spirochete was first demonstrated to be the agent causing syphilis in 1913 by Dr. Hideyo Noguchi at the Rockefeller Institute in New York City, and the use of curative penicillin began in 1943. Is syphilis gone? Hardly. Even with an effective treatment, there were nearly 12 million new cases worldwide in 1999.

Compared with work being done with most infectious agents, there has been lightning-speed scientific progress in the field of hepatitis C. Here's a good word to characterize our advances in understanding hepatitis C biology and the development of effective treatments: breathtaking. Most of us will tell you these days that more than half the patients undergoing hepatitis C treatment are cured. I can't think of another viral infection that even comes close.

But there is always a lag when it comes to the medical system. I might as well cite myself as an example. Unknown to me, in those first days of working in drug treatment, I was looking at hepatitis C in the medical charts of almost every single patient I evaluated. I just didn't see it. Even as 70 percent of new cases of hepatitis C were related to the very patients I treated on a day-to-day basis, I spent those first ignorant months just trying to figure out how to care for patients who used drugs. Even though subsequent testing would show that more than 90 percent of my patients had been exposed to hepatitis C, I was swamped with undiagnosed and unmanaged medical, surgical, and psychiatric conditions that I had been accustomed to referring elsewhere. There were also homelessness, violence, unemployment, and poverty, and the list could go on and on and on. Another reason that hepatitis C is called the "silent killer," as Chris mentioned, is that many other issues make a lot more noise.

But the medical horizon has changed, much as it did for me when I finally realized what should have been obvious: It's hepatitis C, stupid. What happened to Chris also happened to many of my own patients: going to the doctor and getting tested but not getting diagnosed. And even though things have improved, there is still a lot of misinformation out there.

One of the best examples of this is what happened to Chris. "Nope, you don't have it. Your liver enzymes are normal." We know now is that this isn't true, but there are a lot of doctors out there who are still getting this wrong. Because hepatitis C lives and grows in the liver, most people are surprised to hear that only about 15 percent of people with hepatitis C will show abnormalities in their liver enzymes on every blood test. Half the remainder will have liver enzymes that go up and down, sometimes normal and sometimes not. And the rest? Their liver enzymes stay normal, no matter how many times you check them. If you don't specifically test for hepatitis C, you will miss the diagnosis. You just can't tell with the regular blood tests that doctors routinely order, and that's why hepatitis C testing is recommended for anyone with a prior risk factor.

If you make a list of all those individual risk factors, it becomes quite lengthy. But it really comes down to one word: blood. A blood transfusion or organ transplant before 1992, when we began testing the blood supply. Receipt of purified blood proteins, such as clotting factors, before 1987. Long-term kidney dialysis, by way of exposure to other people's blood in the hemodialysis machines. Health-care workers with needlestick injuries, children born to mothers with hepatitis C, and people with HIV. Sexual exposure to someone who might have been infected (who thought to ask?). And, as we've heard, people who have ever injected drugs, including what many consider more mainstream substances, like anabolic steroids and growth hormone, even those who did so only once many years ago.

It is that easy to transmit, when it comes to blood. Actually there is some evidence that intranasal cocaine use and the use of crack-cocaine pipes can spread HCV, via the small amounts of blood that can end up on the straw or the pipe. And also theoretically possible are unsafe tattoos and the sharing of toothbrushes, razors, or even nail clippers, each of which can involve small amounts of blood. I sometimes wonder about people who say they don't have a risk factor: What planet are you from?

When it comes down to this gigantic list of things that might lead to hepatitis C transmission, it is hard to understand the ongoing stigma that can still accompany the diagnosis. It just makes no sense. Plus there are all the ways that hepatitis C *isn't* transmitted. Like hugging and kissing. Sharing eating and cooking utensils or cups and glasses. Actually, even most of the risk factors already mentioned are pretty unlikely to spread the virus. Sexual transmission occurs in fewer than 2 percent of stable monogamous relationships and so condoms are only suggested early in a relationship, or when there are multiple sexual partners or the possibility of another sexually transmitted disease. Mothers pass it on to their children at birth only about 5 percent of the time. And hepatitis C is pretty fragile. It is killed by ordinary household bleach and can't live on surfaces for more than four days. Pure and simple, hepatitis C is just not the kind of illness that should elicit panic. But it is also not the kind of illness you should ignore.

Chapter 2

Understanding

Even though I respected and trusted Rob Huizenga, I thought he was making a big deal out of nothing. "You need to go see a hepatologist," he said.

"A hepatologist? What's that?" I asked, thinking, Why is he sending me to someone that sounds like a snake expert? What I found out was that hepatologists are liver doctors, and there aren't many of them. Focusing on liver disease, especially hepatitis C, is no way to get rich.

Dr. Huizenga referred me to a hepatologist named Dr. John Vierling at Cedars-Sinai in Los Angeles. Dr. Vierling's a big, robust guy, and smart. He reminded me of Santa Claus with no beard and a wall full of impressive medical certificates. When I asked him a question, he'd often start his answer with a laugh. Not a "what a dumb question" laugh, but a "don't worry, I'm ten steps ahead of you" laugh, which helped calm me down.

The first thing Dr. Vierling said to me was, "You've probably had this disease for twenty years"—which was shocking.

"Shouldn't I be dead already?" I asked.

"You could be, but fortunately you're not."

I liked this guy.

As it turns out, hepatitis C isn't the kind of virus that chews holes in your liver right from the beginning. Most of the time you don't see much of anything really serious happening in the first couple of decades after you're infected. But about twenty years in, people start getting the nasty stuff, like cirrhosis and liver cancer. Not everyone does, but if it's going to happen, that's when it usually starts.

"Be straight with me, Doc. Is this thing going to kill me?" I asked Dr. Vierling.

"Chris, hepatitis C can have very serious consequences, but let's not jump the gun. First we have to determine if the virus is still in your blood."

Dr. Vierling ordered another blood test, just to make sure I really had this disease. It turns out that hepatitis C doesn't always stay in your body after you are exposed. About one in four people clear the virus on their own, and even though they don't have the virus in their body anymore, they still test positive. That's because the test only looks for antibodies, which are the footprints of an infection in the past. The trick with hepatitis C is that you have to check to see if it is still around. And if it isn't, you don't have hepatitis C anymore, you don't need treatment, and you aren't going to get sick from it or pass it on.

Naturally, being the fanciful optimist I am, that information steered me back to being convinced I no longer had hepatitis C.

SOBER CHRIS:

I knew it. I'm fine—just the doctors overreacting again. God wouldn't save me from drowning in my drug addiction just to kick me to death on the beach.

JUNKIE CHRIS:

Don't be so sure, man. Shit happens!

Even Sober Chris knew the odds were against me, and that's where they stayed. Dr. Vierling gave me the news: Yes, I had hepatitis C, the chronic active kind, not the good kind that wouldn't adversely affect my body.

But the good news was that I had something called genotype 2, which was easier to treat than genotype 1 and the other strains of the virus. At that time someone like me with genotype 2 had a better than 70 percent chance of achieving a sustained virologic response, or SVR, which means the virus is eradicated from your body. The rate for genotype 1, by far the most common one, would have been less than 40 percent.

So bad news, good news, then more bad news.

"You should have a biopsy so we can get a sense of what shape your liver's in," Dr. Vierling said.

"I don't like the sound of that, Doc. Isn't a biopsy when they cut me open, reach inside, and yank out a slice of my liver?" I asked.

Dr. Vierling laughed his "no problem, I've got it" laugh.

"No, Chris, this is a needle biopsy, where we slide a needle into your liver and remove a very small piece of tissue."

Sticking a long silver shiv into my side and removing a piece of a vital organ, no matter how small, didn't sound like something I wanted done either. I didn't think any part of my liver needed to see the light of day.

Getting those hepatitis C test results is a bewildering experience. First you have it, then you don't. Or maybe you don't, but you probably do. Congratulations, you have the good kind of hepatitis C! But is there really any such thing?

When we look at what Chris went through, it's no wonder that many people are confused. So let's clear some of this up. In the early days of hepatitis C, we had only one test. It was the same test that was developed to screen our blood supply, and it looked for antibodies to the hepatitis C virus as a stand-in for measuring the virus directly. We all get infections from time to time, and our body fights them off. But the infection leaves behind traces of the battle in the form of antibodies. Most of the time these antibodies are useful little proteins, because they can protect us from getting infected again. That is one of the main reasons why we get things like measles and mumps only once.

Checking for antibodies is fairly simple, and so to this day our hepatitis C screening tests still look for antibodies. Today's tests are similar in strategy to the ones that were first developed, but the new tests have become even more exquisitely sensitive. Plus these tests are cheap, relatively speaking. These are all the ideal characteristics of a screening test, and remember, we're using these tests not just on patients but also on each and every one of the fifteen million units of blood donated in the United States every year. Mistakes would be costly, and the dollars would add up quickly.

You could use my own little clinic as an example of how these basic hepatitis C costs accumulate. We have tested about 3,500 people for hepatitis C, because most of the people walking through our door are at risk. Our laboratory charges us eight dollars for each test that we send, which doesn't include our time or the materials it takes to draw and process the blood. It would be on the low side to estimate that the total cost of each of our tests is about twenty-five dollars, because it can be pretty tough to get blood from a long-term drug injector. Sometimes the reality is that there are simply no places left on the arms where you can draw blood. You have to go to a big central vein, such as one in the groin, if you want to get enough blood for a hepatitis C test.

So add in the time it takes to negotiate that procedure with a patient ("You want to do *what*?"), have him or her undress, sterilize the site, and get the blood. Even with the crazy lowball number of twenty-five dollars per test, we're not all that far from one hundred thousand dollars just for hepatitis C screening in my clinic. If those tests were much more expensive, we'd be out of business in no time flat.

Here comes another problem. As it happens, the hepatitis C screening test has one huge weakness: It doesn't actually tell you that you have hepatitis C. It tells you that you were exposed in the past, no more, no less. It surprises many people to hear that something like 15 to 25 percent of people are able to cure themselves of hepatitis C, even without treatment. We don't exactly understand this phenomenon yet, but it appears that the immune systems of some individuals are already primed to kill the virus. After exposure the body's defenses heat up, fight off the virus, and within six months the virus is gone. Period.

But even that successful battle leaves a footprint in the form of antibodies. And that is the Achilles' heel of the test we use to screen for hepatitis C: It can't distinguish the individuals who have the virus from the ones who fought it off. The screening test is positive, regardless. In my clinic more than 95 percent of those tests have been positive, and I almost wonder why I send them. In many settings a positive hepatitis C test elicits alarm and disbelief and is repeated. In my own circumstances it is the opposite. I look upon a negative result with suspicion.

So basically the hepatitis C screening test is just the first step. If it is negative, you are off the hook. But if it is positive it needs to be followed by the kind of test that can directly detect traces of the virus in the blood. These go by a number of names, like viral load or PCR, for polymerase chain reaction. Since up to 25 percent of people who are exposed will clear hepatitis C on their own, about a quarter of people whose screening test is positive will end up finding out that there is no detectable virus in the blood. That is cause for celebration, because it means that you don't have hepatitis C. You cleared it on your own. It is gone, not dormant. If there's no hepatitis C virus around, then it can't damage your liver and you can't pass it on to other people.

Many clinics including mine will double-check, just to be sure that the results are true, just to be safe.

At my clinic we celebrate these negative viral tests, but we celebrate them with caution. One of the concerns about hepatitis C is that a prior infection does not necessarily protect against a new one. More simply said, it is possible to reinfect yourself if you are reexposed. With people who have cleared the virus spontaneously, the evidence suggests that reinfection is fairly unlikely. But we don't downplay the possibility, just in case.

If reinfection were a likely circumstance, then I would see very few negative viral tests in my clinic. The reason is this: Most of my patients have exposed themselves to hepatitis C tens, hundreds, or thousands of different times. The reality of being an injection drug user, particularly before HIV awareness and even now in areas where there is no access to sterile injection equipment, is that a large majority have shared contaminated injection paraphernalia with other people. If you don't have access to sterile equipment, then you will use equipment that isn't sterile. So will the other people you are with, and that is how hepatitis C keeps getting spread around. You don't facilitate drug use by providing sterile equipment, the data is clear on that. But you can stop disease transmission. At least it's a start.

One of the things I always ask my patients during their first office visit is to estimate how many different people they might have shared needles, syringes, cottons, cookers, or rinse water with—any of the injection paraphernalia. Everyone looks away in embarrassment. I think the most common first answer is, "Oh, shit!" But I always make them give a number, even if they don't want to. More than 250 have estimated sharing equipment with at least 100 other people, and almost 50 people have reported sharing with 1,000 or more. If every single new exposure represented a 75 percent opportunity for chronic infection, then none of these patients would be virus-free.

But that is not the case. About a quarter of my hepatitis C patients have had their viral tests come back undetectable, just like patients at every other clinic. It suggests that there is something almost magical about some people's immune systems, in the way they are able to keep hepatitis C from taking root.

There is a tendency to moralize about drug use, and from that derives the belief that, unlike other infected patients, drug users "deserve" to have hepatitis C. But that attitude warrants reexamination, since it is about as enlightened as gloating about a diabetic who has gone blind or lost a leg. That is because a lot of people think that drug addiction is the same thing as drug use or drug abuse. It isn't. Drug use and drug abuse are stupid behaviors, but addiction is different.

You don't become addicted to this or that drug until a deep area of the brain called the nucleus accumbens develops stable neurochemical changes that lead to a compulsion to continue to use that particular drug. There is very good scientific evidence for this. And that means that once you become addicted, it is no longer a simple matter of saying no, much as it is no simple matter to just stop eating and lose that excess weight. The brain says: Do it, I want it, and now I want more. And therefore a drug detoxification program is like a crash diet in both its method and its lack of long-term success: losing the weight is the easy part. Now try to keep every single ounce off for the rest of your life. That is what addicted patients have to do.

For many people, addiction is a lifelong neurochemical harness, not an opportunity to assign blame. That would be like blaming a schizophrenic for acting crazy. And as it was with schizophrenia prior to the development of antipsychotic drugs, addiction will remain an immensely frustrating condition until medical science develops better and more comprehensive medication options. I have all the admiration in the world for people like Chris who have been successful in their recovery. It is truly an amazing achievement. I can't imagine that I would have that kind of strength.

Now we get back to what it means when the hepatitis C virus is detected in your blood. If that is your result, then you really do have hepatitis C. Assuming that the virus has been around for at least six months, the medical term for this is chronic hepatitis C. And that's the situation where you are at risk for its consequences. As you will see, even people with active hepatitis C don't usually end up with the dire outcomes that we always talk about, like cirrhosis, liver failure, and liver cancer, particularly if they stay away from alcohol and take good care of themselves. But it is possible that these things will happen just the same.

The last test that Chris mentioned was the genotype. There are six of them, numbered 1 through 6. The genotype test gives you more information about your virus, kind of like knowing that someone has a pit bull or a cocker spaniel versus knowing only that they have a dog. It is a really important test if you are heading toward treatment. This particular test tells you how likely you are to clear the virus with treatment, how long that treatment should last, and what doses of medications you will need. Chris was fortunate to have gotten the "good" genotype, as if there were any such thing. Basically he had the one that was easiest to clear with treatment, which is genotype 2. Genotype 3 also usually responds well to treatment, but genotypes 1 and 4 are more challenging to get rid of. We know less about genotypes 5 and 6, but they appear to be somewhere in between.

There is more to discuss about these blood tests, and more to discuss about how hepatitis C damages the liver. But enough for now. It is time to move on to the next touchy subject, the liver biopsy. The Dreaded Liver Biopsy, in which, as Chris says, they "yank out a slice of my liver." Nice terminology, Chris.

Chapter 3

Interventions

Being a recovered addict affected my treatment for hep C in lots of ways—good and bad. One of the first things to come up was the whole idea of a needle biopsy. I don't have a fear of needles, as long as I'm the one using them. But other people are using them on me . . . well, that's a different story. I'd already had enough of people jabbing me for bloodwork, and now the doctor wanted to stick this *huge* needle in my body and take out a piece of my liver. I was sure it would hurt—a lot.

Dr. Vierling reassured me, explaining that the biopsy was the only way to get a good picture of my liver and accurately assess what kind of shape it was in. They'd take the little piece of liver gathered in the hollow part of the needle and examine it under the microscope. It was possible that there wouldn't be much in the way of scar tissue, which would mean I wouldn't need treatment. Or the biopsy could indicate that the liver had experienced a lot of damage, and treatment would be necessary.

They'd do the biopsy at Cedars-Sinai, as outpatient surgery, and they'd do it while I was awake. They recommend a pre-op dose of a tranquilizer or painkiller, such as Demerol, and they numb up the area over the liver so the needle doesn't hurt going in.

JUNKIE CHRIS:

Demerol—that sounds good!

SOBER CHRIS:

We don't take drugs anymore, remember?

JUNKIE CHRIS:

A giant needle being shoved into your liver sounds painful.

SOBER CHRIS:

Not gonna happen. No Demerol, period.

When Dr. Vierling was done, I was convinced that the biopsy really was necessary, and it would hurt a lot. Why else would they offer me drugs? The thing is, I don't take anything like that anymore, ever, no matter how hard Junkie Chris pushes.

I began using drugs when I was thirteen. I was in eighth grade, and three of my best friends would get together on the weekends and drop acid. They had been asking me for months, all the way back into seventh grade, to join them but I had always said no. There was this little voice inside me that was telling me that taking drugs was the wrong thing for me to do, and I had been listening to it. But on this fall day in Westchester County, New York, three and a half months after the assassination of my uncle Robert F. Kennedy, my friends asked me again and I said yes. Just like that I said yes, and for the next seventeen years the only thing I cared about was where I was going to get my next drink or my next drug. I went to college and law school, I had jobs at law firms and movie studios in Hollywood, and I even received a master's certification in clinical psychology from Harvard Medical School—but the only thing that really mattered was getting high. I had the craving, and unless you've been there and felt it, you will never understand the obsession and compulsion an addict feels to use his drugs. I describe addiction as similar to dancing with an eight-hundred-pound gorilla, and an eight-hundred-pound gorilla will dance wherever it wants. It will dance in the White House, it will dance in the poorhouse. The point is that if the gorilla wants to dance the addict has little choice. When I got clean and sober on February 17, 1986, that eight-hundred-pound gorilla was locked in a cage and he miraculously went to sleep. When I was dealing with my hep C and was confronted with the decision of whether or not to take Demerol, Valium or anything else for the biopsy or whatever else might come up, the gorilla had been asleep for fifteen years. There was *no way* I was going to wake him up just to take the edge off a liver biopsy.

A few years before I began contemplating how I

might deal with the painful procedures, muscle aches, sleeplessness, and whatever other by-products of treatment for hep C I might encounter, I was working on the daytime soap *All My Children*, and my back went out in a serious way for the very first time. For a whole week I was in excruciating pain. I couldn't get comfortable for a second, and I could barely walk. I couldn't change my clothes without help. The crew at ABC had to dress and undress me on set. During the week I stayed at my mother's Manhattan apartment while my wife and kids stayed at our house in Westchester County. One morning I woke up at my mother's place in crippling pain. It was so bad I could barely breathe, but I still had to get dressed and go to work. The only one around to help me was my mother, so I went to her room. She was sitting in bed, reading the newspaper, and when she heard me she looked up and said, "What's wrong with you?"

I said, "Nothing, Mom," and shuffled back to my room. I had to lay my clothes on the floor and kind of squirm into them to get dressed, but I did it and I got to work.

That whole week I never took painkillers. I figured if that hadn't sent me back to drugs, the biopsy wouldn't either.

So we schedule the biopsy and I show up at the hospital, totally sober and totally scared. There are all these other people there, waiting for their biopsies, and they've taken whatever it was the doctor was offering. They're stretched out on gurneys, narcotized and pretty happy about the whole thing, while I'm sitting there in my hospital gown, trembling with fear and anxiety.

JUNKIE CHRIS:

I think you might have made a mistake not taking the drugs, man!

SOBER CHRIS:

Om Nama Shivaya, Om Nama Shivaya. . . .

JUNKIE CHRIS:

What are you doing?

SOBER CHRIS:

Saying the mantra. It'll help us get through this.

JUNKIE CHRIS:

The only thing that's gonna help is a shot of Demerol.

SOBER CHRIS:

Not an option, buddy.

When it was my turn they took me to the exam room, Dr. Vierling came in, walked around behind me, told me to hold my breath, and *boom!*—it was done. I was amazed at how fast it was, at the fact that it was nothing like what I'd been dreading. It just felt like a quick jab, a kidney punch. I know there can be complications, like with any surgery, but for me it was absolutely nothing.

After the biopsy was over I remember thinking, Well, that was the worst of it, because I was absolutely certain that there was nothing wrong with me. I'd only done the biopsy because, as usual, the doctors were overreacting. The results would show what I already knew—my liver was fine, I was fine.

The liver biopsy is always a big deal, even though it usually isn't much of a big deal at all. The thought of being stabbed with a needle long enough to reach an internal organ is daunting enough, and then there's the idea that it could hurt a lot and you get to be awake to find out if that is going to be the case.

But from a medical standpoint, the liver biopsy really is a fundamentally important procedure when you have hepatitis C. That is because it is the single most reliable way to determine if you actually need treatment. Imaging studies like ultrasound and CT scanning can help with that decision, but they offer only a rough overview of what is going on. And there are new blood-testing and imaging strategies that are beginning to get more accurate in terms of their ability to predict scar tissue. But nothing measures up to biopsy, at least not yet.

Why do we care? The main reason is that many people with hepatitis C don't actually need treatment. After having the virus for twenty years, only about 15 to 20 percent will have cirrhosis of the liver. That's it: only 15 to 20 percent. But for those who do get cirrhosis, it's a big deal. "Cirrhosis" is the medical term for a lot of scar tissue in the liver, enough to encircle and isolate the islands of liver cells so that they can never completely regenerate. You have probably seen pictures of a liver with cirrhosis, pebbly and gristly and yellow. That is the scar tissue taking over.

A lot of people don't know that if you cut out half of a healthy liver, it will regrow in a month or so. I suppose that's not a topic that usually comes up in casual conversation. The liver is amazing in its ability to regenerate but there are limits to its resourcefulness; even the healthiest liver can't penetrate scar tissue. So if you have cirrhosis, even if it is from hepatitis C and you are successful at getting rid of the virus, the liver will never return to its former healthy state. So it is important to gauge how things are going in terms of scar tissue development. If you are headed toward cirrhosis, it's time to consider getting treated for hepatitis C.

We don't have very good noninvasive ways of predicting the progression of liver damage because we have only begun to understand how the liver damage from hepatitis C takes place. As it turns out, hepatitis C doesn't really do much to damage the liver on its own. It is a peaceable virus that inhabits about 10 percent of the cells of an infected person's liver. Accrued liver damage is not related to the rampaging hepatitis C virus but instead occurs from the immune system's attempts to purge the liver of infected cells. In some people, the immune system reacts vigorously to hepatitis C virus infection. If that kind of immune attack is aggressive and ongoing, you will develop a lot of scar tissue and even cirrhosis, much as you will have a bigger scar on your skin when a wound becomes infected and inflamed.

The flip side is that some people's immune systems basically ignore hepatitis C. For many infections that would be disastrous, but for the amiable hepatitis C virus it works out great. No battle, no scar tissue, no problem. People like this can have hepatitis C for decades and have a perfectly normal-looking liver. Gerard Wallace is a peer educator at my clinic, and he has had hepatitis C for more than forty years. His liver biopsy showed no scar tissue whatsoever.

This leads us to two last points about the hepatitis C virus, trick questions I like to ask people who attend my program. First, which genotype damages the liver the most? And second, how high does your viral load have to be before you worry about your liver? Almost everyone gets these wrong at first, but it's not so hard to answer them correctly if you remember that hepatitis C itself doesn't cause the liver damage.

The answer to both questions is, it doesn't matter. Genotype and viral load don't predict liver damage from hepatitis C. The hepatitis C virus doesn't damage the liver so the genotype doesn't help predict that. Some genotypes are harder to get rid of but they all have the same tendency to elicit an immune-related attack.

Similarly, the hepatitis C viral load is simply the result of an interplay between the virus and the immune system; the liver is more of a bystander. Most of us are more familiar with the HIV model, in which a high viral load elicits alarm. It is different with hepatitis C. Believe it or not, when you have hepatitis C you make over a trillion new virus particles every single day—no wonder you're tired, right? The immune system clears away most but not all of them, and what is left behind is your viral load. It is just your particular number.

A high hepatitis C viral load doesn't mean there is a lot of liver damage and so there is no reason to do serial tests to see if the number has changed. I have some patients with severe cirrhosis; they have low viral loads because there is very little liver left to host the virus. On the other hand, I have many patients with perfectly healthy livers and viral loads in the many tens of millions. This is another reason we have to rely on the liver biopsy to help sort things out.

Basically the liver biopsy starts when a small amount of local anesthetic is injected into the skin and tissue over the liver. Everyone is hoping to hear the words "general anesthesia" at this point, but that would be disastrous. The texture of the liver is a lot like tough Jell-O. It has to remain still in the brief moments when the actual biopsy occurs, otherwise it could be torn. Since the liver moves up and down a bit when you breathe, you have to be awake enough to hold your breath for a few seconds.

Once the local anesthetic has taken effect, the liver biopsy is performed. It is quick. You are told to stop breathing, and then, in less than an instant, the biopsy is done. There is a benefit to this speed, much as it is actually easier to have a Band-Aid yanked from a wound, despite the unease it creates beforehand.

Sometimes the biopsy is done in one quick pass if the needle is long enough, or sometimes it is taken in a few separate passes if a biopsy gun with a shorter needle is used. Then it is over. Since you can't hold a piece of gauze to your liver to stop it from bleeding, you have to put pressure on it by lying on your right side for a time. That is the boring part, but at least the biopsy is over.

Does it hurt? It can, but it usually doesn't hurt much. I know you're thinking that this is some kind of doctor-speak minimization, kind of like hearing "just a tiny pinch" before the burning spear is rammed into sensitive flesh. But in fact this is exactly what I have been told by my patients. The reason is the liver itself does not contain nerves that convey pain, but it is covered by a skin, called a capsule, which does. That is why people with hepatitis C sometimes say their liver aches—they are feeling their swollen, inflamed liver stretching the liver capsule, a sensation that is uncomfortable. That same capsule will tell you that a needle is passing through, and it will also complain for a few days about the small amount of blood and swelling that will be left after the biopsy is over. But for most people this level of discomfort is far less than the worry that they put into planning for the big event.

But it is true that some people's biopsy experiences are worse than that. In my clinic the number of patients who return to say it was painful is on the order of one in twenty. Often they had more significant scarring than we anticipated, making the actual passage of the biopsy needle more challenging. In others it related to inexperience on the part of the person performing the procedure. That is why I like to keep my liver biopsy referrals to a single place, where they do them every day.

And last, there can be complications. They are uncommon, but they do happen. Mostly the issue is something like bleeding around the liver that may even require a transfusion, or poking a hole in some nearby structure that wasn't meant to be touched. Out of hundreds of biopsy referrals, I have had one patient that needed a transfusion. Two others had holes poked in their breathing muscle, or diaphragm, which drapes over the top of the liver. Naturally one was my staff member, Larry Galindo, but he ended up with only a small temporary air leak and so he was able to go home later in the day. The other patient who had her diaphragm pierced ended up with a partially collapsed lung, and then she needed a chest tube to reinflate it. That wasn't good because the chest tube hurt and she had to stay in the hospital for an extra day, but after that she had no further problems. Well, that's not exactly true. If you can believe it, the hospital had the nerve to bill her for their own mistake, and she had to spend time dealing with that ridiculous problem. Another of my patients brought me his liver biopsy report from a different hospital, which came back showing "normal cartilage." Basically, it meant that they missed.

There are rare reports, something like one in two hundred thousand, where people have died. Although this would not happen in experienced hands, and no one that I know has ever seen this happen, this is the very thing that scares many people off. But realistically it is the most important reason to recommend a liver biopsy judiciously. A liver biopsy is only useful if it will have an impact on the decision to treat, or on how aggressively to approach treatment once it begins. If the results will have sway, then the liver biopsy has value. If not, then it is simply not needed.

Persuading my own patients to have a liver biopsy can be a challenging task. I don't blame them for their ambivalence. After all, many have had bad experiences within the medical system, and so it is not an environment they trust. Doctors sometimes incise drug abscesses without anesthetic to teach addicts a lesson. Pain medications are severely limited or even withheld after big operations because they might lead to addiction. Drug users with painful problems like broken bones are accused of drug-seeking, even though they're just looking for a little relief. On several occasions I have had patients with cirrhosis go to the emergency room because they had built up toxic levels of ammonia in their blood, a condition called hepatic encephalopathy, which is caused by liver failure. They were sick, confused, and disoriented, but were promptly discharged from the emergency room without testing. "You're just loaded," they were told.

A trusting relationship helps melt my patients' fears. They know that they can reach me and that I will help them if the biopsy goes awry. I am especially lucky to have many patients who have already gone through the experience, for good or for bad, and are willing to offer up their knowledge and support to others. That goes a long way toward easing the apprehension.

I am also fortunate to have good peer educators. One that I already mentioned is Larry Galindo, who had his diaphragm punctured during his biopsy. Although I know of no kinder or more considerate an individual, Larry spent many screwed-up years as an addict, drug dealer, and prison kingpin; many patients in my community who have never met him are familiar with his reputation as a tough, ruthless badass. You would think that being shot and stabbed on five separate occasions might have immunized Larry against the fear of a little liver biopsy, but that wasn't the case. Mr. Tough Guy still likes to tell people that when he had his liver biopsy, he was so nervous that he actually bent the bed rail all the way over. He is still on the record books as the only patient who has ever broken a stretcher like that, badly enough that they had to send it off for repairs. No wonder his diaphragm was pierced.

One of the best things we did at my clinic was to make a video of an actual liver biopsy.

My staff member Gerard, whom I have already mentioned as having had no scar tissue in his liver, had a biopsy that he allowed us to tape. The biopsy was performed by Dr. Alex Monto at the San Francisco VA Hospital. Chris McNeil, who is responsible for the many amazing hepatitis C educational videos that have come from my clinic, did all the taping and editing. The video is remarkable for its brevity and uneventfulness. Whenever I have shown it to patients, they ask one question: "Can I see it again?" After they do, the fear is gone and we are able to move forward. I had to nag Gerard for more than a year to get him to narrate it, but finally he did. It is now posted with our other educational videos on our clinic's Web site, www.oasiscliniconline.org, where I hope it is doing some good.

I had no fear at all once the biopsy was over. There was no way in the world I could believe there was anything wrong with me because—I *felt* fine. My experience of hepatitis A and B was that they laid you out and made you want to die, and I didn't feel that way at all now. The doctors kept asking me about symptoms, and the only one I had was fatigue.

SOBER CHRIS:

Yeah, I'm fatigued. Find me somebody in their forties, with kids, a job and a life, who isn't fatigued.

JUNKIE CHRIS:

Hey, man, if you have this hep C thing, just imagine how you're going to feel if you treat it and get rid of it—you're going to be like Superman!

SOBER CHRIS:

I don't have it. I'm tired, that's all. I feel fine. There's nothing wrong with me.

I walked out of Cedars-Sinai, went home, and got on with my life, without an inkling it was about to implode.

From the outside, the life I went home to looked great. My wife, our three kids, and I were living in a perfect little house on a perfect little street in perfect little enclave near the beach. But there were major problems underneath, and they were about to surface.

We'd spent several years in New York, during my stint on *All My Children*, until I realized that doing a soap means you're dead in the movie business. I went back to LA to get my movie career going again, but when you're dead in Hollywood, resurrecting yourself can take a while. My kids were getting older, school fees were adding up, and there just wasn't enough money in the bank. So I was looking around for other ways to make a living: in finance, the Internet, and television production. And as much as I cared about my wife, I knew our marriage needed to end. We had been married for almost fifteen years and despite the bonds of our kids and our history together, we had grown apart.

Looking back on it, I think that when I got sober I began a search to find myself. Joseph Campbell said, "The privilege of a lifetime is being who you are." But because of my addiction and the extraordinary circumstances of my life I had abdicated myself to a lifestyle and a paradigm imposed by external considerations. In my recovery I have followed a path of self-discovery, often selfishly, and that took a huge toll on my marriage. Although I didn't realize it at the time, I wanted to leave but just didn't know how to do it.

So all of this is going on in my life. I have lots to think about, and before I know it six weeks have gone by and I haven't once thought of that nice Dr. Vierling, the long needle he shoved under my ribs, or what he might have found hiding in my liver. I'm driving home from a meeting or something, and I'm wondering why I've never heard back about the biopsy.

SOBER CHRIS:

You never heard back because everything is fine and the good doctor figured you didn't need to be told that.

JUNKIE CHRIS:

Or maybe he got busy and just forgot to tell you that you have cirrhosis.

I pull into my driveway, and before getting out of the car I call the doctor's office, just to make sure everything is copacetic. The nurse answered, and as soon as I identified myself she said, "Oh! Mr. Lawford, I'm glad you called. We need to get you in for treatment right away!"

"Treatment for *what*?" I said.

"For your hepatitis C." That's when I panicked.

I got Dr. Vierling on the phone, and in a classic bad-news doctor voice he said, "Come in right away. We have to talk about your results and what we're going to do about your treatment."

Hearing "your treatment"—in that split second, I knew my life was about to change dramatically. I sat in my car, looking at the house, where my wife was watching tennis and my kids were playing computer games, all blissfully unaware of my unfolding predicament. I noticed the serene ordinariness of my neighborhood, the predictable beauty of the Southern California afternoon, and I felt the anxiety and fear of a life-altering transformation. Nothing had changed, but everything was different.

JUNKIE CHRIS:

I knew it! Karma is such a bitch.

SOBER CHRIS:

This isn't a punishment, asshole.

JUNKIE CHRIS:

It's karma, man. All those years you spent as a dope fiend—did you really think the universe was going to give you a pass?

SOBER CHRIS:
Play the victim if you want. I'm going to look at it as an opportunity!

JUNKIE CHRIS:
Yeah, right—an opportunity for what?

SOBER CHRIS:
We'll see, won't we?

The biopsy showed that I had focal bridging fibrosis, which means there is scarring of the liver tissue that jumps from structure to structure. It's often a sign that you're headed for cirrhosis of the liver. Now, I knew what cirrhosis was, and I knew I didn't want it. My father died of cirrhosis when he was sixty, and he was yellow when he died. I've seen cirrhosis up close, I know what it is. It is a nasty, painful way to die. I also knew that the farther down that road you go the less likely it is that your liver will recover. The liver is an amazing organ and it can regenerate itself, but past a certain point, it's difficult. Past another point, you die.

Dr. Vierling also mentioned my viral load, which really wasn't meaningful to me. I mean, six million, three million—millions of something is not good when you're talking about something bad. What got my attention was not my viral load, but the fact I had bridging fibrosis, which could lead to cirrhosis. That I understood. I remember one of my friends described a cirrhotic liver as a piece of cardboard, with that dry, crumbly texture. I kept imagining my liver going from this big, plump, juicy organ to a chunk of cardboard. It wasn't a comforting image.

When someone has looked at your liver under the microscope and sends out an alarm, it is a warning that will catch your attention. That is something I depend upon. The liver biopsy is the single most reliable piece of information for determining whether or not you need to be treated for hepatitis C. I have patients in all stages of mental, physical, and psychosocial disarray, a daily reminder of my own good fortune. My job as their doctor is to determine whether or not they need this challenging, potentially lifesaving hepatitis C treatment regardless of any potential barriers. It is my ethical duty. I rely upon the liver biopsy to accurately and reliably advise me of this need. If a patient needs treatment and there are other issues that may create problems, such as drug use or depression, then my priority is to ensure that these issues are addressed. "You don't have to die of hepatitis C," is what I tell my patients. "You can if you want, but you don't have to." That is something I believe.

I was never trained to interpret liver biopsies. Once I finally recognized the gigantic hepatitis C problem I had on my hands, I began referring patients to local gastroenterologists for biopsy and hepatitis C treatment. I probably don't have to convince you that my patients were not exactly welcomed with enthusiasm. In any case that was neither their expectation nor mine. But I did expect my patients to benefit from the additional level of expertise that the specialists could offer.

Unfortunately that didn't happen. I guess it was too much to ask at the time, because not a single one of my patients was offered anything more than a "Don't worry, you're fine" opinion. No biopsy, nothing. It was a fruitless and frustrating exercise. But once I discovered that my own hospital's radiologists had begun doing liver biopsies, I became their first best customer. Then I had to learn how to interpret the reports.

Fortunately that is not particularly difficult. The most important thing a liver biopsy tells you is how much scar tissue there is in your liver. The medical term for scar tissue is "fibrosis." There are different scoring systems for this, but a common one rates the amount of fibrosis from 0 to 4. You know what 0 means. But if you have stage 4 fibrosis, it is exactly the same thing as saying you have cirrhosis. It is the highest level of liver scarring that you can have. In Chris's case he had what is called bridging fibrosis. On the fibrosis scale that would be a 3. Not quite cirrhosis, but a lot of scar tissue nonetheless.

The other characteristic that is examined is called inflammation, which is the redness that accompanies any wound you get. Again, this is given a score, from 0 to 4. If you have a cut on your arm and it becomes red and inflamed, it is more likely to scar—in other words, develop fibrosis. The same is true of the liver. If there is no inflammation, fibrosis formation will proceed slowly if at all. But if the inflammation is aggressive, then the fibrous scar tissue will develop more quickly, increasing the risk for advanced fibrosis or cirrhosis.

Once you understand these things, it becomes easier to see how a liver biopsy report can be used to guide a treatment decision. Many people want to know what fibrosis level indicates that treatment is needed, but there is no single answer to a question like this. As one example, I may recommend hepatitis C treatment for a young person with minimal scar tissue because I am anticipating the development of more significant liver damage in the coming decades. I probably wouldn't make the same recommendation for people in their sixties with the same biopsy results, because they are unlikely ever to develop enough liver damage to cause problems. I was once referred a healthy ninety-two-year-old man who had hepatitis C and stage 2 fibrosis. I congratulated him on his longevity and sent him on his way. Some things just depend.

It can also be helpful to know when the initial infection occurred, because then it is possible to estimate the speed of progression. For instance, if you have had hepatitis C for twenty years and you have stage 2 fibrosis, then it is taking about ten years for you to advance one stage, and it will be something like another twenty years before you get to stage 4 fibrosis, or cirrhosis. That can be a relief. My patients rarely know exactly when they were infected, but injection drug use is such an efficient way of transmitting hepatitis C that about half are infected in the first year of using drugs with a needle. That gives us a useful way to estimate the duration of hepatitis C infection: We just subtract one year from the duration of needle use.

With all the important information you get from a biopsy, why doesn't everyone get one? Well, nowadays, as hepatitis C treatment becomes increasingly effective, many doctors do not hesitate to offer treatment to those who are very likely to be successful, such as those who have easy genotypes to cure or who are early in their infection. I suppose I could needle Chris at this point (sorry, Chris, pun intended) by mentioning that with genotype 2, he would probably fall in this category and might reasonably avoid biopsy altogether.

Sometimes the history, physical examination, and blood tests indicate that the liver disease is advanced and in that circumstance a biopsy is unnecessary and could be dangerous. A biopsy is pointless for people who have decided they want to be treated regardless of the amount of liver scarring, perhaps because they have severe fatigue or another medical condition that gets worse because of hepatitis C, or because they just want to get the villainous virus out of their body. Others need no biopsy because they refuse to consider treatment under any circumstances. Then for some people—such as many of my own patients—there is the expense: The cost runs to thousands of dollars, and not everyone has insurance that will cover it. In that situation, it is perfectly reasonable to make the treatment decision on the basis of a good history, a physical, and blood tests.

I still recommend liver biopsies when I can. Even under the best of circumstances, many of my own patients will have significant challenges with staying the treatment course. It is especially important in my setting to make sure that any decision to offer treatment is sound. Because hepatitis C does not progress all that rapidly in the majority of patients, we generally find that treatment is actually needed in fewer than 20 percent of those we see.

Chapter 4

Decisions

Wen I got to Dr. Vierling's office to talk about treatment, he explained what the protocol would be, and that it would be a long-term thing, over a period of months. HCV is a virus that hides, millions and millions of cells disguising themselves to evade your natural immune system. The main weapon against it is interferon, which is the same thing your body produces to fight viruses. When it was first discovered, lots of people thought it might be the cure for cancer, just an incredibly powerful drug that would do amazing things. Interferon also makes you feel terrible, physically. When you have the flu, it's not the virus that gives you all those terrible aches and pains; it's the interferon. The injected form of interferon floods your system with far more than you can produce naturally, so it's better at spotting and taking out invaders, like HCV. The earliest treatments for hepatitis C used straight interferon, which you had to inject every couple of days or even daily. Pegylated interferon maintains its level in the bloodstream better, so you inject it once a week. The standard treatment also includes ribavirin, which is another antiviral. If interferon is the tire iron you use against HCV, then ribavirin is the steel-toed boot. It doesn't kill the virus directly but it kicks it in the nuts and slows down its reproduction.

You take the interferon and the ribavirin and you go in there swinging and you kill a bunch of these bastards, but it takes a lot of swings of that tire iron and that boot to get them all. If you stop the treatment too early, there may be a clump of virus hiding somewhere. Then, once the antiviral drugs are out of your system, the virus comes back stronger than ever. And the fact is treatment doesn't work for everybody—like my two friends, who had endured months of interferon and still had HCV at the end of it. Since then, the treatment had become much more effective, but there was always a chance that it wouldn't work. How big a chance I was about to find out.

JUNKIE CHRIS:
I knew this wasn't going to work. Might as well get high.

SOBER CHRIS:
We're not getting high. We'll just take it a day at a time and trust . . .

JUNKIE CHRIS:
Yeah, I know . . . trust God. Right. . . .

Dr. Vierling explained all this to me, and then he said, "You're lucky, Chris, because you have genotype 2. We mostly see genotype 1, and that's much harder to treat. You have a better than 70 percent chance of a good outcome."

SOBER CHRIS:

Those are pretty good odds.

JUNKIE CHRIS:

There's still a 30 percent chance that you'll go through this torture and it won't work.

Then Dr. Vierling said, "Look, even if it doesn't work for you, your liver will get a year off from fighting the virus, and that will help you. Right now your liver is getting bombarded by this illness all day, every day, but once you start treatment, your liver will get a vacation."

One of my friends told me a few days later, "If you have any cancer cells or any other bad shit in your body, the interferon will take 'em out." I wasn't sure my friend knew what he was talking about, but I was willing to hold on to anything that made treatment more palatable. Even if it wasn't true—and I found out later it's not.

JUNKIE CHRIS:

Okay, I'm on board with wiping out hep C and maybe killing cancer cells, but eleven months of that sounds expensive.

SOBER CHRIS:
I wouldn't count on the cancer cells.

JUNKIE CHRIS:
Whatever. The point is, these drugs can be pricey. You think our insurance will cover it?

SOBER CHRIS:
I have no idea. We'll figure something out.

B e on guard for fanciful ideas from helpful friends and from places like the Internet where accountability is questionable. If interferon searched out and destroyed latent cancer cells, then we'd all be taking it and the disease of cancer would be on its way to eradication. It's true that interferon in high doses is used to treat a couple kinds of cancer. But unfortunately there's no collateral cancer benefit to hepatitis C therapy, aside from reducing the risk for liver cancer when the treatment is successful.

F ortunately, paying for treatment became a nonissue when Dr. Vierling said, "We might be able to get you on one of the clinical trials at Cedars-Sinai." I had heard of clinical trials. I thought they had something to do with using experimental drugs on people who were so sick they had no other choice, but it was free and that sounded good to me. I later found out that clinical trials are crucial to testing not just new drugs but new combinations and ways of using old drugs. The trial I participated in would determine the length of protocol for future hep C patients with genotype 2. Today it makes me feel really good to know that my eleven months of treatment helped demonstrate that a six-month treatment protocol works just as well.

In my advocacy I've learned a lot more about treatment cost and reimbursement. I've found that paying for medical care is a major hurdle for the four million plus who have been exposed to hepatitis C and may need treatment to overcome it. But at the time I didn't have any idea how lucky I was to get treated for free. I actually felt like I was doing Dr. Vierling a favor: "Oh, you need a guinea pig? Well, okay."

I know it's always worth researching your options, even though that's not what I did. My friend Bill helped me through my treatment and then, maybe a year after I was done, he was diagnosed with hep C and started treatment, so I was able to pay him back. Unlike me, Bill researched anything and everything about hepatitis C treatment, and he chose to be treated at the Veterans Administration clinic in San Francisco. Turns out the VA treats more hep C patients than anybody else; they interact with the Centers for Disease Control on research, and they're a great option for anyone who's eligible. But I wasn't since I'm not a veteran, so I'm glad Dr. Vierling was able to include me in the study.

Even with the treatment being free, my feeling was, Okay, we're going to punch you in the face for eleven months but we're not going to charge you for it. I was still reluctant to begin treatment—primarily because I basically felt fine, and this treatment was going to wreck the quality of my life, my ability to function. I really believed that once I started treatment, I'd be sick and miserable and on a couch, unable to move, for eleven months. I'd already been through this as an addict, when to get better I had to take myself out of my life for ten days or thirty days in treatment or detox, and I just didn't want to do that ever again.

Another reason for my reluctance was that I'd be tied to a hospital for eleven months, and I did not like hospitals. I guess nobody does, but hospitals fill me with dread and fear. All my experiences with hospitals had come about through some drug-related screwup—mine or a loved one's. I associated hospitals with a part of my life I'd left behind and didn't want to go back to. They brought back too many memories, all of them bad.

And I already had plenty of uncertainty to deal with in my professional life, without adding treating my hep C to the mix. I was trying to get this new thing going, producing political segments for an entertainment-news show, and applying for jobs at financial firms while praying my dot-com would take off and make me rich. My paycheck was coming from the good folks at *Extra* who figured they might be getting access to my Rolodex of celebrities to meet their never-ending demand for high-profile fluff and scandal. I thought I might actually learn how to produce a short TV news segment and use those same celebrities to talk about issues that mattered.

While I was working on a segment for *Extra* I attended the Republican convention in Philadelphia to do a piece on celebrity advocacy. That convention had major consequences for the country, and me. The Republicans nominated a guy who would do his best to destroy much of what's best about America, and I met a woman—I'm going to call her Carrie—who provided me with a deceitful, inappropriate bridge out of my marriage. Carrie and I started an affair, and a short time later I left my wife and moved into a hotel room. Actually I spent a few weeks more or less living in my car. I drove around with my toiletries, my yoga gear, and an extra pair of jeans, with my suits for *Extra* hanging in the backseat. I'd park in front of my old house, trying to get my kids to come out and talk to me, then I'd give up and drive to Carrie's house, and sometimes I'd crash at the hotel. After a couple of weeks of that my cousin Maria Shriver offered me a place to live.

She and her husband owned this house nobody was living in on a beautiful street in Pacific Palisades, right below Will Rogers Park and close to where my kids lived. They'd bought the house from a guy who'd been a star on a big TV show in the eighties but had fallen on hard times. The place had been vacant for a while when they bought it. They'd let it sit there for a few years while they decided what to do with it, and by this time it was in bad shape, pretty much a teardown—a three-million-dollar teardown, because this is Pacific Palisades, but a teardown nonetheless. It was a big, rambling place, with a pool, a giant tennis court, and a crumbling wall surrounding the grounds. The house had the feel of Boo Radley's place in *To Kill a Mockingbird*—overgrown, ramshackle, and spooky. I remember always being cold because a lot of the windows were broken, so there was a draft, and the heat didn't work. The stairs and balconies were in disrepair, and the place hadn't been cleaned for years. My kids hated it because there were spider webs everywhere. Maria didn't know what she was going to do with it and she told me, "Stay there until you put your life back together." My friend Hiro gave me some of his old office furniture, I bought a bed, and I moved in.

The second night in the house, I met the mouse. Carrie was with me in the master bedroom, and we heard this squeaking.

"What was that?" Carrie said, pulling the covers up around her.

"I don't know," I said. "There are so many weird noises around here, it's like we're living in the woods."

"Go find out," she said.

"How am I going to do that?" I asked.

"Get out of bed and look. . . . Please."

I figured the noise had something to do with the way the house creaked, or the overgrown branches that scraped up against the outside, but I got up and looked around anyway. I'm a sucker for a woman in any kind of distress. And there in the brick fireplace was this little mouse, standing up on his hind legs, his little front legs in the air, doing that whisker-twitch thing with his nose, looking right at me, and squeaking like he was trying to tell me something.

"Look, baby, it's a mouse." I said.

"A mouse! What's a mouse doing in the bedroom?"

"I don't know . . . he probably lives here. He's cute."

Mice don't bother me, and I don't bother them. Live and let live has always been my credo at times like this.

"Can you get it out of here?" Carrie asked.

"How?" I don't have a huge amount of nurturing or empathy in me, but the little I have wouldn't let me scare or hurt a mouse.

"Open the door and see if it will leave," she said.

I opened the door to the balcony, which had a stairway down to the yard, and just went back to bed hoping the mouse would take the hint and leave. I kept an eye on the door and finally after about an hour, he walked out to the balcony and was gone. It saddened me to see him go. He wasn't a bother and he seemed friendly. I needed some friends, even the four-legged variety.

Two days later he was back in the fireplace. He showed up there three or four times a week, after I'd gone to bed. I never saw him in any other part of the house, only in the fireplace. Of course, that fireplace was never used for anything but a mouse-house. He'd come visit and I'd say hi and talk to him for a little while. Later on, while I was on the interferon, I'd rant at him and he'd just stand there, twitching his nose and listening. It was cheap therapy for me.

So that's where I was—separated from my wife, my work situation unstable, living in a dilapidated house, and talking to a mouse. I figured I had no emotional resources available to deal with eleven months of treatment for hep C, which I wasn't sure I needed anyway, and that affected the way I heard everything Dr. Vierling said. I was looking for any justification not to initiate treatment. So when he told me I was on the downside of the fibrosis progression slope—that on a scale of 1 to 4, 1 being the best and 4 being the worst, I was between a 2 and a 3—what I heard was, "You're a 2. That's not so bad." I asked Dr. Vierling what was likely to happen if I didn't get treatment. How sick would I get? How fast? Could I stay at 2 or 3 for the rest of my life? Or would I be dead in three months? He said—and this is true, and it's one of the frustrating things about this disease—that there's no way to predict any of those things. Each person has his or her own course of this disease, and we just don't know how it'll play out.

SOBER CHRIS:
There has to be an alternative to treatment. There has got to be a better way to take care of this.

JUNKIE CHRIS:
Yeah, man. . . . You know all those smart people at the drug companies are working their asses off on this. There's a big market here. They'll come up with a silver bullet in no time.

I'm sure glad I didn't listen to Junkie Chris, because he was wrong. The current treatment is pretty much the same as what I had in 2001, and the best estimates are that the cure rates may increase 10 to 20 percent in the next five years. There is no magic bullet, and there's not going to be one anytime soon. But I didn't know that, and I didn't want to know it. I was looking for any reason at all to *not* deal with the fact I had this disease. If you'd told me that I could cure my hep C by sprinkling fairy dust into my hair, I would've held on to that.

And nobody can lie to you better than you can lie to yourself. When Dr. Vierling told me, "There's a very good chance you'll continue to get sicker, but there is the possibility that the disease won't progress," all I heard was the "but," and I convinced myself that I just didn't need treatment.

I went back to Dr. Huizenga, my internist, and I was telling him about my decision and all these reasons why I didn't want to start treatment and why it made sense that I didn't start. He sat there and he listened to me very impassively and then finally he said to me—with a little bit of impatience and maybe just a touch of anger—"Listen to what you're saying! You've got a better than 70 percent chance this treatment will work. Do you know how many people would give their right arm to have those odds of curing a life-threatening illness?"

That's all he said. That's all he needed to say. I hadn't really gotten it up to that point—the severity of this illness, the chance I had for a full recovery, the opportunity I was being given and how I was about to throw it away.

SOBER CHRIS:
Hey, remember the last time you did things your way?
You stayed sick for fifteen years. Maybe you should
do it differently this time. Listen to the man, he's a
doctor!

So I decided to initiate treatment.

I am fortunate to work with a physician's assistant named Amy Smith; she has a kind and gentle way about her and possesses the sort of remarkably level temperament that makes her a favorite with some of our most difficult patients. She never complains when that works against her. She and I regularly see new patients referred for hepatitis C because there are not that many places in our area where you can get the disease treated. A lot of doctors simply don't want to do it. Although I have already spoken a great deal about taking care of marginalized patients with hepatitis C, we see our fair share of "regular" hepatitis C patients as well. It doesn't matter to Amy and me how you got it, we treat everyone the same regardless of their background. The virus has the same approach.

But there is a particular advantage to taking care of addicted patients. Most come to our clinic having family, friends, or acquaintances who have been diagnosed with hepatitis C, had a biopsy, or even had treatment. They often have some of the same freaked-out attitudes about hepatitis C that Chris has described, but at least they are oriented toward reality. The same is not always true of the other patients.

"I see that you were referred for hepatitis C," I'll say. At this point I'm usually looking through their papers, fruitlessly trying to find blood tests that either weren't sent or were never done. "Yes, I am here to get treated," they'll respond. That is when I know we are probably in trouble, and now is the time I am going to find that out: "Great! What can you tell me about the treatment?" "Not much. My doctor sent me here to get treated." That is a typical response but not the one I hope for. It is an answer untainted by reality.

When people find out they have hepatitis C, they figure,

Well, now I have to get rid of it. These days we have become so accustomed to antimicrobial treatments that our first consideration is to take a pill to make it go away. But despite the amazing progress in the development of medications to treat hepatitis C, it is just not that simple. Hepatitis C treatment can be remarkably effective and it appears to cure more than half the people who complete it, but it is not to be undertaken lightly.

Hepatitis C treatment generally consists of two medications. As Chris mentioned, the backbone of treatment is interferon, which is administered by injection under the skin, and it is usually combined with ribavirin, a medication given orally as a pill. These medications are typically taken for six to twelve months or sometimes longer.

Interferon is actually a family of natural substances made and released by the body's white blood cells in response to certain infections, such as the flu. It was discovered in 1957 by Dr. Alick Isaacs and Dr. Jean Lindenmann, who never received the Nobel Prize but probably should have, and it was named for its ability to interfere with virus reproduction. Interferon is an immunologic clarion call, summoning the immune system to attack. When given in sizable doses as it is in hepatitis C, it enhances the immune response to the point where many people who have been chronically infected can eliminate the virus from their liver. It is now available in a long-acting form, called pegylated interferon. The letters *peg* stand for polyethylene glycol, a molecular carbohydrate chain that envelops the vulnerable interferon molecule, protecting it from degradation and allowing it to remain more stable in the tissues. Instead of injecting regular interferon three times per week, which was standard for many years, a weekly injection of pegylated interferon is now the norm. This form of interferon has improved treatment success rates from 40 percent to 55 percent, a big advance.

That is the good news. The bad news, as Chris already mentioned, is that interferon is in part responsible for the marvelous way you feel when you have the flu. As a by-product of its beneficial effects, interferon also causes fever, muscle and joint aches, and a host of other physical and mental annoyances. There will be more on this later.

Ribavirin is interferon's antiviral accomplice. It was first synthesized in 1970 by Joseph Witkowski, a chemist at ICN Pharmaceuticals, and first approved as an inhalant for children with respiratory syncytial virus (a common viral infection of the airways) after having failed to achieve approval as a treatment for the flu. It was subsequently found to have activity against hepatitis C when used in combination with interferon, and it was approved for that use in 1998.

Although its exact mechanism of action is not entirely clear because it does not work alone against hepatitis C, ribavirin has the effect of doubling the efficacy of interferon treatment. Unfortunately ribavirin comes with its own set of issues, the biggest of which is hemolytic anemia, a kind of anemia in which the red blood cells explode. Unlike other anemias, it does not respond to iron or other supplements and the onset can sometimes be dramatic. This is one of the reasons why regular blood testing during treatment is so important, because if you don't detect the hemolytic anemia early enough, it may become so severe that treatment will need to be stopped.

Having said all this, I hope that you are getting the picture of hepatitis C treatment as a physically and mentally significant intervention, one that will last from twenty-four to forty-eight weeks or maybe longer. It is chemotherapy in the purest sense, as interferon is also used for kidney cancer and melanoma, a kind of skin cancer. It requires regular and sometimes aggressive monitoring for drops in blood counts and many other problems. It is not just something that you show up and take.

I didn't know any of this when I started referring my patients for liver biopsies. That was a point at which I still had some small hope that there would be a place to send my patients for hepatitis C treatment. But because this came at a time when hepatitis C treatment for drug users was not recommended, some part of me knew better. I had become familiar with the impact of stigma and prejudice on the care my patients received when I referred them elsewhere. It made me protective. As for hepatitis C, it made me want to learn more.

In 1998 the landmark paper on the use of interferon and ribavirin to treat hepatitis C was published in the *New England Journal of Medicine*. The article was on my desk when a drug representative from the Schering-Plough Corporation named Stacey Coates showed up at my office. I have never figured out how or why she found me—an addiction doctor entirely unschooled about hepatitis C, in a crummy office in a decrepit building in the middle of a disorganized old hospital campus. She asked me if I treated hepatitis C. I said no. Then she asked me if I would be interested. I looked at her in disbelief, and thought about it for the briefest of moments. There was really only one possible answer. "Yes," I said.

Chapter 5

Initiation

O nce I made the decision to start treatment, it was important for me to figure out exactly what was going to happen. Back then hep C wasn't nearly as visible as it is now. Now you go to a recovery meeting and there are people who are dying from liver cancer caused by their hep C. Some are looking for liver donors, and many are talking about their treatment. This was not the case in 2001. But I still came across some horror stories about the treatment. I heard about a guy, a recovering drug addict, who ended up relapsing on painkillers, and then the interferon made him so angry and crazy that he started a fight with a state trooper who'd pulled him over. He almost got shot, and he did get thrown in jail. I didn't want to go to jail, and I sure as hell didn't want to relapse on drugs.

And there was someone else who simply didn't get off his couch for eleven months. He just lay down and didn't get up. That scared me more than anything. I move fast in my life. "You can't hit a moving target" has always been one of my credos. Good or bad, I wasn't slowing down for anyone or anything. I grew up in a family where the ethic was always to suck the marrow out of life, to live life to its fullest, and you do that by doing. There was a large part of me that believed that if I wasn't active, wasn't accomplishing things, I would die.

"That's not going to be me," I swore.

I heard these stories about people who go crazy, kill themselves, relapse on drugs, break up their marriages. That is the truth about what can happen to some people who get treated for hep C, especially addicts and alcoholics, though most people get through treatment without these levels of difficulty. But being an over-the-top addict/alcoholic, I stayed focused on the more dramatic outcomes. In my consultations with my doctors I tried to get them to be very specific about what was going to happen, and they couldn't. All they could say was, "We can never predict how these medications are going to affect people. Sometimes we think this person will never be able to do it and they sail through it without a problem. Some people just can't tolerate it at all."

None of it was very reassuring.

My family makes it a point to shake off physical illness. Case in point: In May 2008 my uncle Ted Kennedy had a series of seizures and was diagnosed with brain cancer. The doctors sent him home from the hospital with orders to take it easy. First thing he did was take his sailboat out. I love my uncle Teddy! When I was a kid and I was sick, it wasn't so much a lack of sympathy: "Stop whining! We don't want to hear about it." It was more like: "There are much bigger problems in the world than yours, and you're either part of the solution or you're part of the problem." And I don't necessarily disagree with that. I'm not saying that the ethic of not complaining and just forging ahead is a bad thing. But it doesn't serve you very well when you have to go through something like this. You've got to have a balance. There has to be some nurturing in there somewhere. That's not something I ever got, and I ended up believing I don't deserve it.

So when I was diagnosed with hep C and started treatment, I told myself that this was my business, my thing to deal with, and I'd get on with it. I really did not reach out to my family for support; I did not include them in my treatment at all. I didn't tell my mother about the diagnosis and the treatment because by then, she was dealing with her own illness. I didn't reach out to my wife because, for one thing, she was angry at me, and I also felt like I'd dragged her into enough of my crises already.

I didn't sit down with my kids and tell them about my illness, about the treatment, about what might happen. I felt they were too young. David was thirteen, Savannah was ten, and Matty was three. Plus there was already so much upheaval in their lives that I didn't want to throw something else into the mix. But more than anything I honestly didn't think my family had any kind of stake in this thing. I was the one who was sick, I was the one who had brought this on myself, I should be the one to deal with it—on my own. That was how I was conditioned to approach illness. Looking back on it, I see now that my family had a huge stake in my hep C. It could have killed me. They should have known. I should have told them and included them.

I asked my son David, who's now twenty-one, if he remembers me telling him about the hep C or if I included him at all in what I was going through in treatment, and he said, "All I remember is that you were angry all the time and you always blamed it on the medicine you were taking."

David was right that I was angry during treatment—so angry, in fact, that I ruined my credit because every time I got a bill in the mail I would get so mad at whoever sent it that I'd say, "Screw you and your bill!" and just not pay it. One of my good friends in recovery used to greet me every time we met with, "How you doing today, Chris? That interfury you're taking still kicking your butt?"

The isolation fed the anger and the anger fed the isolation. It was like a vicious spiral and it was the wrong way to do things.

Finding support in this disease is absolutely crucial and the obvious place to go to for support is your family or your partner. Well, all I had was a girlfriend I hadn't been with for very long. At first I had this insane idea that I should just not tell her that I had hep C. I remember thinking, Oh, my God. Maybe she'll break up with me. Maybe she'll never have sex with me again. Maybe she'll overreact. But I did tell her.

"Carrie, I have something I need to talk to you about," I remember saying to her.

"What's the matter?"

"Remember a couple of weeks ago I went to the doctor and he tested me for HIV and hep C?"

"Yeah," she said as if she knew I had AIDS.

"Well, I don't have AIDS."

"That's good."

"But I do have hepatitis C," I said.

"What's hepatitis C?"

"Well, it's a blood-borne disease that affects your liver."

"Is it contagious?" she asked.

"Not really. Unless we shoot up together and use the same needle," I said, trying to be funny.

Carrie wasn't amused.

"What about sex?" she asked

"It's more likely you would get it from my toothbrush than from having sex with me," I said. I was repeating a line I thought I'd heard from one of my doctors, but I wasn't 100 percent sure it was true.

"Hmm," she said. "Better keep your toothbrush to yourself."

Carrie and I had a difficult relationship, partly due to the circumstances under which we came together and partly due to our personalities. There was a lot of emotionality between us, and she found ways to drive me crazy, but she also helped me deal with the situation in ways no one else ever had. For one thing she had the attitude that it was important to be fully present and conscious, to think about what I was going through and what I was going to do about it. That was new to me. When I was using, I had always approached difficulties with the attitude, "The less conscious I am, the better." Recovery had introduced me to the benefits of awareness, but I still had a long way to go in that area.

Carrie also made it clear that she wanted to be a part of my treatment. She came with me to the hospital in the beginning, which I'd never let anyone do before, but after a while she lost interest due to the deterioration of our relationship, her self-involvement, and my increasingly disagreeable nature. In the past I'd always dealt with my medical issues on my own, both because that's the way I was brought up and because most of the time they were self-inflicted. When you end up in the hospital because of a drug overdose and everybody's standing around your bed going, "Jesus, what are we going to do about you?" for the fourth time—you start segregating that part of your life from the people who are still in your life.

And I still had some shame and guilt around hepatitis C, because I saw it as self-inflicted damage. Even though it was a by-product of my addiction and even though I knew addiction is a brain disease, it was difficult for me not to blame myself. I kept thinking, Fifteen years later, my drug use is screwing up my life—again. My treatment of my hep C was, for the most part, a lonely and isolating experience partially caused by my perception and partially by the treatment itself. I remember sitting on the bed, getting my medicine, and my needle ready to inject the interferon into my body, not really knowing what effects it would have but expecting the worst.. I felt very much alone and alienated from the world in general and the people in my life in particular.

It is easy to fall into the mind-set of believing the cure

is worse than the disease. If you do that you'll stop treatment because the cure is hard. It is a hard thing, but it's also the cure, and it's possibly going to rid your body of a life-threatening virus. I was really clear about that. That was the overriding thought that got me through the treatment protocol, and it saved my life.

Hepatitis C has a remarkable tendency to create upheaval. From an outside perspective the process of coming to a treatment decision may sound simple. But you might be surprised to hear how intimidating it can be. One of the first patients I focused on was Ron. He was in his early fifties. After decades of heroin use he had finally gotten on methadone and stopped using drugs, allowing me to start him on antidepressants and get his diabetes and high blood pressure under reasonable control: He was a success. He was also one of the first patients whom I diagnosed with hepatitis C, and one of the unlucky minority who had developed cirrhosis, something I didn't need a biopsy to tell me. It was clear he needed to be treated.

We made an appointment to discuss referral to a gastroenterologist. That morning I briefly caught sight of him in the waiting room, but when I went to bring him into my office he was missing. I saw another patient, but afterward Ron still wasn't there. That wasn't like him. I asked if anyone had seen him, and someone said that they thought he was in his truck. Sure enough. Not *in* his truck, exactly, but unresponsively draped over the side of the truck bed like a human sack of grain, half in and half out. Stressed out just by the idea of hepatitis C treatment, he had taken four 10 mg Valium tablets and gone outside to distract himself from reality by rearranging the junk in the back in his truck. Then he fell asleep, sort of standing up.

Before I started treating hepatitis C, my experiences were not always this unusual, but they did tend to coalesce along these lines. Part of it was my patient population. But the bigger part of it was my failure to recognize the immensity of what it means to be told you need hepatitis C treatment. Coming to understand this was a big factor in my decision to learn to treat hepatitis C myself. My patients did better with special handling, and they weren't going to get that elsewhere.

The other factor was my utter failure to convince other doctors that my patients needed to be treated for hepatitis C. It wasn't as if I were referring active drug-using homeless schizophrenics. My referrals were handpicked. They were patients I liked. They almost always showed up on time, and I was managing every other medical and psychiatric condition that they had. But not all doctors can see through the background to the person inside. They found every excuse to avoid offering treatment, and there were many excuses to be had.

When Stacey Coates from Schering-Plough materialized in my office, I had just lost a patient to liver failure. I made her put away her hepatitis C treatment glossies because I already had a copy of the main research article and I don't like that stuff anyway, but I did hit her up for a package insert. In a twisted medical way those can be a really good read if you are able to see the microscopic printing. The package insert is the information that the company puts together under the direction of the FDA. It has all the bad with the good, and references to boot. I wanted to learn everything there was to know about the bad.

There was no shortage in that department. I was familiar with interferon's tendency to lower the white blood counts and the platelets. I could handle those problems and the hemolytic anemia and the thyroid disorders and the potential for infections and heart problems and worsening of lung disease. I had been well trained in years past. But there was a lot more to hepatitis C treatment than that.

My concern was more along the lines of what would be medically categorized as interferon's "neuropsychiatric toxicity." That term is a shortcut for a gigantic list that includes significant conditions like depression, mania, and psychosis. It also includes other problems effects like insomnia, irritability, anxiety, fatigue, and confusion, to name a few. I had patients who started out with these kinds of difficulties, and it was clear from what I read that they would have the tendency to get worse. I was hoping to avoid reading about my hepatitis C patients in the newspaper.

My patients also had a tendency to develop alternative strategies for dealing with problems of this nature that eventually got them in trouble. The benign term for this would be *self-medication;* what it really meant was that by offering a toxic treatment, I could put my addicted patients at risk for relapse. And addiction is far more lethal than hepatitis C.

Carrie was conscious about taking care of herself. She approached issues of self-care from a vantage point I had little familiarity with. For instance, she knew how much I hated hospitals, hated even being there, so she said, "While you're at the hospital, build a cone around yourself, a cone of light, so you're protected from all the bad things you associate with the place." I had never been in a hospital surrounded by a cone of white light before. I found it to be very therapeutic and empowering.

I tend not to plan ahead about much of anything. I make a decision and then I go forward without a lot of thought or mental preparation. Carrie had a different approach.

"What is your intention with this treatment?" she asked me.

"What do you mean, 'intention'?"

"What are you going to get out of it, and how?" she said, as if it were something obvious to consider.

"I want it to work and get rid of the virus," I said.

"What else?" she asked.

"I don't know what else," I said, feeling a little defensive.

"Well, maybe you should think about it."

I'd never really thought about intention before. I decided to be very specific about what my intention was when it came to the treatment of my hepatitis C. I saw that time in my life as my forty days and forty nights wandering in the desert. I believed my life was on a razor's edge—on one side was death; on the other was transformation. My overall intention was that this experience would be a transformative one—not just physically but emotionally and spiritually. On a more micro and pragmatic level I broke down the overall intention of transformation into five specific intentions.

1. I'm not going to use drugs or alcohol.
2. The treatment is going to work for me.
3. I'm going to complete treatment.
4. I'm not going to kill myself.
5. I'm not going to kill anybody else.

I held on to those five intentions. I took them seriously, and over the next eleven months, I came back to them again and again.

The issue of safe sex did come up again, of course, and we did *not* practice it. The doctors had told me that HCV is not as easily transmitted as HIV. My understanding was that HCV is not present in semen, just in blood, so you have to have blood-to-blood contact during sex for the hep C virus to be transmitted to your partner. So, transmission through sex is really, really difficult unless you're having bloody sex, which we weren't into. I held on to the line, "You could transmit this easier from a toothbrush than you could from having sex," even though I wasn't totally sure of that. I felt like this was a disease I got because I used needles, and as long as I wasn't using needles, I wouldn't pass it on to anybody else. Carrie checked with her own doctor, but like most internists he knew very little about this disease. So she decided to trust mine. We never used condoms, even though I couldn't say, "I can't possibly give this to you." Because there is a chance.

I was also nervous about what the interferon and ribavirin would do to my ability to have sex. I'd heard the drugs could be debilitating to one's sex drive. I mean, who wants to have sex when you're sick, tired, and depressed?

JUNKIE CHRIS:

You do, man. A little fatigue or depression never quelled your desire for sex, but your ability to perform might be another matter. If it were me I'd get some insurance.

SOBER CHRIS:

Viagra.

JUNKIE CHRIS:

That stuff will keep you going even if you're dead! Make sure you get the doctor to make it refillable.

Let's go over those risk factors one more time. The word to remember is blood. Toothbrushes are a potential transmission risk because of blood from bleeding gums, but in truth the risk is more theoretical than real. In fact, I know of no documented case of hepatitis C related to a shared toothbrush.

On the other hand, we do know for sure that sex can transmit hepatitis C. It is uncommon, but it does occur in nearly 2 percent of stable monogamous relationships. And Chris's understanding about the virus not being present in semen is untrue: Hepatitis C has indeed been detected in semen, albeit at low levels. For this reason, the CDC says that condoms are not necessary in long-term relationships, but they are recommended early on in relationships and for persons who have multiple sexual partners or sexually transmitted diseases. Remember, even though the transmission risk is low, there are far more sexually active adults than drug injectors. That is why a sizable fraction of persons in this country with hepatitis C, about 15 percent, are thought to have contracted it through sex.

As I said before, it will make the entire treatment experience more tolerable if you include people who will support you in the process, and you go through it together. There can be this temptation to keep the treatment secret because it can be almost invisible. There are some physical effects, but it's not like all your hair falls out. You could probably go through the whole protocol and not let anyone know, but it really should not be done that way. The treatment itself is alienating enough, and trying to do it all on your own will make you feel like a pariah, that there's something terrible and unacceptable about you. Couple that with the mental and emotional side effects of the medication, and it's deadly.

I was constantly questioning if I was doing everything I was supposed to do, in the right way. The stakes were so high, and I didn't want to screw it up, do anything wrong. It's hard to mess up because the shots of interferon are preloaded, but I was still afraid that somehow I'd make mistakes and jeopardize my treatment. After a while the constant questioning of myself began to wear on me.

I really think that's the biggest thing I learned through all of this. My orientation toward illness was just to take care of it, and to take care of it alone. Don't talk about it and don't complain about it. Just go get it done and stop whining. What I learned is that that attitude can be useful, even admirable, but it's not always the best way to treat yourself. Certainly not with a disease like this, because it's so demanding and debilitating, physically and emotionally. Again, I believe strongly in intention. If your intention is to defeat this disease, and you surround yourself with people who love and support you, then your chances of maintaining your intention are much greater.

I wasn't able to do that with my family, but I did find support in my recovery groups. The fact that my disease came out of addiction meant there was a commonality of shared experience with other addicts and alcoholics. These people are my tribe. If I'm feeling crazy and scared, I know if I pick up the phone and talk to another addict or alcoholic, they're going to get it. No judgment, no "Why don't you just stop?" I'm going to hear, "Yeah, I get it. You're doing great. Just keep doing what you're doing, a day at a time." There were friends who were with me 24/7, throughout the whole thing, whenever I wanted them. Always answered the phone. Always came over when I asked. Whatever I needed, they were there for me without hesitation. My friend Bill virtually moved in with me to keep me from becoming isolated, my buddy Kale put up with my endless self-examination and worry, and my friend Andrea would stay on the phone with me for days listening to me rant about my crazy girlfriend. That's the nature of recovery. I had that kind of fellowship and support when I was newly sober, and I had it again when I went through my treatment for hep C. It was the same kind of life-or-death situation; my friends in recovery showed up for me like my life depended on it—and it did.

These friends didn't just keep me company and listen when I needed to vent, they reminded me on a daily basis of the principles for living my life I'd learned in recovery. These reminders were enormously helpful in terms of the day-to-day struggle of getting through treatment. One day at a time. Turning it over. Believing in a power greater than myself, one that would do for me what I couldn't do for myself. Believing that there's some real purpose to this ordeal, that good will ultimately come out of the experience, and that while it may not look like what I imagine, it will be exactly what I need. Believing pain is the touchstone of spiritual growth, and no matter the outcome I would receive something of great value in the process.

There was only one time when I didn't get that unconditional support, but it turned out okay in the end. This was at a recovery support group I went to regularly, and it was one of those days when I was just unbelievably angry, sick, and tired of the whole thing. The way this group was set up, instead of raising your hand to talk, you got called on. The guy running the group—this big, musclehead biker—called on me and I just went off. You know: "I don't want to be here. I don't like any of you people. As far as I'm concerned you're all full of shit." I just went on this five-minute rant. I didn't want anybody to tell me anything or say anything to me or try to make me feel better. I just wanted them to leave me alone.

I'd been coming around to these meetings for fifteen years, and I'd learned that, left unchecked, my angry isolation could blow up my bridge to recovery and it wouldn't be long before I was drinking and using again. One of the basic principles you learn in recovery is that the way to keep what you've got is to give it away. You reach out to somebody new or somebody who's struggling to stay sober and say, "Here's my number, call me if you want to talk," even if it's the last thing you want to do at that moment. There was a newcomer at the recovery group meeting, with something like twenty-five days sober, and afterward he was talking to the guy who'd been running the meeting. I went up to the newcomer, and I said, "Hey, man, my name's Chris, and I want to give you my number. If you're having trouble staying sober, give me a call." And the biker guy looked at me and said, "You know what, Chris? He doesn't need your number. He already knows how to be angry."

JUNKIE CHRIS:

What an a-hole. You're not going to take that, are you?

SOBER CHRIS:

I am kind of angry.

JUNKIE CHRIS:

If you can't vent in a recovery meeting, where are you supposed to vent?

SOBER CHRIS:

Maybe he's right. I feel like I'm losing it. If people in recovery think I'm out of line, maybe I am.

JUNKIE CHRIS:
That guy was out of line. Those rooms have to be safe.
You can be as crazy and angry as you want to be as
long as you don't use.

I told the guy, "Screw you pal, and the horse you rode
in on." And I gave the newcomer my number anyway and
I left.

You know, on the one hand the muscle-head biker was
right. But on the other hand the wonderful thing about
those mutual support groups in recovery is that you can
go there and tell everyone how you're really feeling and
not get judged for it. I was judged, and that was not what
I needed. In that moment I was an angry asshole, and I
really needed a place where it was safe to be an angry asshole.

A few weeks later the guy came up to me and apologized. He said, "Man, I was wrong to say that to you."
That really helped restore my sense of having a place to
go where I could be as angry or as depressed as I needed
to be and still get support. That's the only time I got that
kind of judgment, and, in his defense, the guy had no idea
what I was going through. I was not one of those people
who raised my hand and said I was going through hepatitis C treatment every time I shared in recovery, because I
did not want the attention. Don't get me wrong; I was full
of self-pity, and I wanted support and understanding from
the people I was closest to. I just didn't want public attention and public scrutiny. Besides, it's not like I had nothing else to talk about. There was a lot of drama in my life

that was a lot more interesting to me than my treatment protocol.

What I realize today is that it's very powerful for people who are going through treatment for hep C to have other people who've already been through it share their experience publicly. If I could do it differently I'd share more than I did about my treatment. Looking back, I think there was a part of me that was just in denial, and that's why I wasn't being more open about it. And that made the whole thing much harder, on me and everybody around me, than it needed to be.

The idea of a support network was not something I initially had much interest in. It doesn't really fit into traditional medical training, in which medications and interventions dominate. It was only in caring for addicted patients that I began to see its power.

Then I met Dr. Don Kurth. He was an addiction psychiatrist and the incoming president of the California Society of Addiction Medicine, an organization I belonged to. He was openly in recovery and had an amazing story about it that he would share with anyone who would listen. I got to talking with him about his recovery, and he asked me if I had ever been to an Alcoholics Anonymous meeting. Having been in the field for a number of years, I was kind of embarrassed to admit that I hadn't. So he invited me to come to one.

If you are not a part of the recovery community, you may have a skeptical attitude about AA or Narcotics Anonymous or the other branches of like-minded recovery programs that have sprung up using a similar model. I know I did.

Don't these things just amount to a bunch of people who get together to talk about not drinking, not using drugs, or not doing something else they want to do? So what? Admittedly my skepticism had already been tempered by a body of medical evidence that the AA model of recovery is at least as effective, if not more so, than any other behavioral intervention. But my personal biases persisted. I am not an easy sale, but that attitude was entirely transformed in a single hour. I was blown away by the honesty, the generosity, and the universal support. The participants rose up through their connectedness. They left with the strength to fight on for another day.

No one in that room will remember I was there, save for Dr. Kurth. But what they did on that day was change my entire approach to taking care of hepatitis C in the patients who weren't supposed to be treated: people with addictions, mental illness, homelessness. Some patients would be straightforward, but not these, and I was becoming skeptical of my ability to integrate the kind of education and support they would need into the hepatitis C treatment process. I was already having trouble keeping up with the education part because I had so many patients with hepatitis C, and of course I wanted to avoid the spectacle of more comatose patients in my parking lot. But more important, I had already had enough patients die of hepatitis C. The ones who were dying tended to be the kinds of patients who would need an additional layer of support. I decided to harness the power of community to help my hepatitis C patients, so we could help one another.

Some people in recovery think that if you're sober, you shouldn't take antidepressants, and I don't agree with that. I don't have anything against antidepressants for anybody who needs to take them, but *I* don't want to take them. For one thing I want to experience every aspect of my life as fully as I can. I mean, I'm an actor. I'm all about experiencing things, good and bad. And I'm also a guy who spent a large part of his life on a couch, narcotized, and I don't want to go back there. I want to be fully present all the time.

Depression is a very common, well-known side effect of the interferon/ribavirin treatment for hep C, so Dr. Vierling offered to start me on antidepressants as we initiated the protocol, and I said no. Before Dr. Vierling mentioned it, I hadn't ever heard of antidepressants as part of the hep C protocol. Now I think it's standard. Months into the treatment, when I reached a point when I felt like I needed antidepressants, I went to Dr. Vierling and asked for a prescription but it was too late. It can take several weeks for these drugs to ramp up and become effective. By that time, I'd only have a couple of months left on the hep C protocol, and then it would take another month or so to taper off the antidepressants. I decided the pills just didn't make sense for me.

When my friend Bill went through his treatment, he took Paxil. He told me that getting off the antidepressants was as bad as the treatment itself. I figure it was just as well I didn't take anything.

Initiation

I would like to interject: Interferon can make you nuts. In the best of worlds it can make you edgy and irritable for the six to twelve months or more that you are on it. In the worst of worlds people have killed themselves, killed other people, or gone completely off the deep end. Time and time again I hear, "I don't want to take one of them nut pills." But if the side effect of treatment were nausea, an itch, or a rash, or whatever, wouldn't you take something for it? I would expect so. That is the very reason you might need to take something to help your mood: because interferon is going to screw it up.

My patient Bob had a history of bipolar depression. Within two weeks of starting hepatitis C treatment he told me, "I have never felt better in my life." Right. I have since learned to hate it when people say that, because as I soon discovered, Bob was on his way to an acute manic crisis and ended up at the local psychiatric hospital after about fourteen weeks of hepatitis C treatment. He was given a couple of new psychiatric medications, and some months later when he was stable we tried hepatitis C treatment again. This time the mania took about twice as long to manifest but the same thing happened: off to the John George Psychiatric Pavilion he went. But because Bob had significant and advancing cirrhosis, we decided to try one more time. We waited a couple of years and worked really hard on getting his medications right. It wasn't easy but now he's cured. He's cured of hepatitis C because of those nut pills. They saved his life.

There's a certain amount of prep work before you start the protocol. For instance, I had to learn how to inject myself. Considering how many needles I'd stuck in my arm, I thought that was kind of odd. But I'd only ever shot up intravenously so I had to learn how to give myself a shot under the skin, in the thigh.

I was worried I wouldn't be able to keep up with the protocol. I'm not a regimented, structured person in general, and I had never been sick to the point of having to do something every single day for weeks and months. The closest I'd come was getting on methadone, and that's easy. You show up at the clinic, they give you a dose, and you drink it.

This was much more complicated. You have to inject the interferon weekly and take the ribavirin pills twice a day. Every month you go to the hospital to get bloodwork done. In the eleven-month protocol they checked my viral load at the third month and the sixth month, but there were other things they kept track of monthly. For instance, interferon can affect your production of red blood cells and cause serious anemia, so they monitor that. When you get your blood test, they give you the meds for the next month.

I really worried about how I was going to keep track of what I was taking. Would I remember to take the ribavirin like I was supposed to? And as it turns out, that can be a problem because one of the side effects of the treatment for me was confusion and memory problems. I was nervous about getting the dosage wrong. I worried about losing track and taking too little, not too much.

See, my orientation through this whole process was, I am killing this virus. Maybe I watched too many cartoons as a kid, but I pictured the hepatitis C virus as these purple-and-black furry animated bugs with giant teeth, millions of them, racing through my body and ravenously taking bites out of my liver. And when I injected the medicine one of them screamed, "Interferon! Run for your life!" and interferon swarmed through my body stomping to death a whole bunch of the little bastards. But one of the little bugs is sneakier and smarter than the others and hides from the interferon and never gets killed. *That's* the one I wanted to get. That was what I cared about. I thought that if I missed a dose, that could be the dose that would have taken out the sneaky bastard that was hiding in my spleen or in some remote corner of my liver. I was obsessed with making sure I took my medication when I was supposed to, so there was no escape for the virus.

There's a lot of preparation, all these decisions to make, and finally, I get to the night when I take my first interferon injection. I knew I was about to begin something that was going to take up to eleven months of my life, and I had no guarantee it was going to work. I'd made the commitment to myself that it was going to work, that I was going to get to the other side, and I kept focusing on that, but the truth was I was terrified.

Much of my initial terror was around the anticipation of how sick I was going to get. I was most afraid of the physical effects but it turned out that the mental stuff was far more challenging, but, fortunately, I didn't know that then.

I remember going home to my teardown, where my only friend was a mouse, and I was so aware of the fact that my life was in ruins, in every respect: my family life, my professional life, all of it. I laid out the pre-loaded syringe of interferon and the two ribavirin pills and I said, "This is it. This is the beginning of my forty days and forty nights. I'm either going to transform, or die." Then I stuck the needle in my thigh, swallowed the pills, and waited for something to happen.

When I'm scared I have to *do* something. When my first kid was born, I was thrilled but I was also terrified. I went home and I washed every window in the apartment. As soon as I injected the interferon and took the ribavirin, I had this unbelievable urge to move furniture, so that's what I did. I decided to move the television upstairs to the bedroom. This was before everyone had flat-screens, and the television I was moving was massive, a giant Sony Trinitron that must've weighed more than a hundred pounds. It had taken four of us to carry it into the house, but I got it upstairs by myself. It was like those stories you read about people so scared they lift up the front of a car.

As soon as I got this TV upstairs, I panicked. I was convinced that if I kept the television there, I'd never leave the bedroom, and I'd turn into that guy who stayed on his couch for eleven months, so I carried it back downstairs. I was so exhausted I lay down, and I noticed that—nothing had happened. I didn't feel any different. Finally I fell asleep.

I woke up in the middle of that first night feeling like something strange, unpleasant, and powerful had entered my body, but it wasn't until twenty-four hours later that I felt the full effects of the drugs. A nasty, creepy, clammy, achy, flulike sickness enveloped me, draining my energy and plunging me into darkness. After a day or so of this misery I started feeling a little better. Each day the effects lifted a bit until I felt almost normal, and then it was time for the next injection.

That's how it went every week, for forty-eight weeks.

There is a tendency to want to rush into hepatitis C treatment: It seems that once you've made the decision, it should be the time to dive in. Most of the people I have seen with that attitude have underestimated the misery they are about to undergo and overestimated their ability to endure it. They are setting themselves up for failure. This was something I learned from the first hepatitis C patients I treated, and this was something they came to learn from one another. If you were going to run a marathon you would train for it. The same is true of hepatitis C.

I had selected a group of five reliable and interested patients who needed hepatitis C treatment. I was lucky to have a large group from which to choose. Earl, Phil, Linette, and Cinnamon already had cirrhosis; Mary had bridging fibrosis, like Chris. They recognized my lack of experience but preferred it to the kind of condescending expertise they might have encountered from specialists at places they didn't even have access to.

We started with the education basics. This five-on-one

business was good for me, far more interesting than repeating the same thing five times over. We initially talked about the liver and the virus, about transmission and how to avoid it. We talked about the importance of avoiding, or at least reducing, alcohol consumption: Our mantra was "alcohol and hepatitis C are like gasoline and fire." We talked about the fundamentals of hepatitis C treatment: interferon injections and how to do them, ribavirin and how it was taken by mouth twice daily, in doses of four to six pills based on genotype and weight. How to determine treatment duration: twenty-four weeks for the "good" genotypes 2 and 3, and forty-eight weeks for the rest.

We discussed treatment monitoring. Blood tests would be taken on weeks 2 and 4 and every four weeks thereafter, to monitor for reductions in blood counts and a host of other potential treatment-related problems. The first viral test would be done at twelve weeks, and if the virus had not declined by at least a hundredfold by that time, the chances of a successful treatment were only 2 to 3 percent. But if it had declined by that amount or was undetectable at treatment week 12, then that was called an EVR, or early virologic response, the beginnings of a positive treatment outcome—but no more than that. They came to understand that the absence of detectable virus during treatment or even at the end of treatment was only a measure of hope, not success. Our holy grail was the SVR, or sustained virologic response, which meant that there was no detectable virus six months after the treatment was over. More than 90 percent of people with an SVR would never see the virus again and were probably cured.

Of course we also talked about the basics of side-effect management. How drinking fifteen to twenty eight-ounce glasses of water daily was the very best way of helping with side effects, but no one knew why. About the importance of even a small amount of exercise, even when getting out of bed was a major task. The discussions were unstructured, based on questions and concerns. They were interactive and positive. They were evidence based. There was no fearmongering.

Earl and Phil agreed to start treatment first, and they both had genotype 1. Within twenty weeks all five had begun their medications. It was a committed, bedraggled, wonderful bunch, and an experience that convinced me we were here to stay. I filed the organizational papers for our new nonprofit community-based medical clinic, Organization to Achieve Solutions in Substance-Abuse (O.A.S.I.S.). Later, after many potholes and stumbles and mistakes, we would become a recognized leader in the treatment of hepatitis C patients with addictive disorders. But at this point, we were still just propping one another up.

Chapter 6

Continuation

During my treatment I spent a good amount of time in the Cedars-Sinai hepatology waiting room. There was usually someone there who was totally yellow: another person with advanced liver cancer. There were lots of people waiting for liver transplants or dealing with a liver transplant. They were glad to be alive, but honestly it did not look like a life I wanted. Still, it might be something I'd have to face.

One of the things I learned during this process was that if you have hep C, a liver transplant is not necessarily going to save your life. First of all, a transplant is unbelievably expensive. It usually takes a long time to find a suitable donor. Baboons are not an option. You have to get on a list, there are no guarantees that a liver will become available before your number is up, and if you're lucky enough to get a liver there is a chance your body will reject it. You have to take antirejection drugs for the rest of your life, and that compromises your immune system. The surgery leaves you with a really big, really ugly scar. Here's the real kicker: Getting a liver transplant doesn't mean the hepatitis C virus won't come back. And often, when it does, it comes roaring back with a vengeance and it can make you cirrhotic in a few years and kill you soon after.

Even so, as a last resort, a transplant was always at the back of my mind.

SOBER CHRIS:
Worst case, if this interferon thing doesn't work I'll just get a new liver.

JUNKIE CHRIS:
Great, then you'll be sitting in here looking like these people.

SOBER CHRIS:
At least I've got options.

JUNKIE CHRIS:
No, you've got the list. What if you're number nine million on that list?

That is what went through my head, sitting in that waiting room.

It's interesting, the subject of liver transplantation. Ten thousand people die in the United States each year from hepatitis C, our number one reason for liver transplant. Unfortunately for every person who gets a new liver, something like four people die waiting for one. It is a huge, difficult surgery, and removing your liver will not cure your hepatitis C: There is more than enough virus in the blood to infect the new liver. Your new liver will probably get cirrhosis much faster, and you'll need to take hepatitis C treatment anyway.

So if treatment is offered, don't fool yourself: Transplant is not a better option. New medications will improve hepatitis C treatment outcomes in the future, but interferon will be with us for a long time. It's going to get better, but easier? Probably not.

These may be good facts to have on hand, but for my patients liver transplantation is hardly ever an option. The problem is, the kinds of patients I see aren't listed for liver transplants. Sometimes there are good reasons like psychosocial instability, but more often it is for uninformed and prejudicial reasons, such as the fact they are taking methadone or have a history of mental illness. Our little treatment group was finally fighting back, though. Five patients limping through hepatitis C treatment, and me, stumbling through the medical management, all of us focused on curing the virus and making liver transplant irrelevant.

We met for one hour each week upstairs at the clinic. There was lunch. At times people could be grumpy or irritable or just plain sick; that was to be expected. But we kept things positive. Each would discuss his or her previous week, for good and for bad. Every week I taught them something new about hepatitis C, choosing some aspect of it that we'd just heard in the introductions. They ate it up, eager to understand what was happening to their bodies. With five people on treatment, we faced a cornucopia of problems; we checked out rashes, thinning hair, canker sores. No one person had all the problems, and that ended up being helpful: "Thank God I don't have *that*." Treatment milestones were shared. Something would always come up that I didn't know, and I'd look it up for the next week. At the end of the group I would draw blood for whatever tests were indicated.

One of the things that wore on me was that it seemed like I was never able to get definitive answers to my questions. It wasn't that the doctors and nurses weren't willing to answer questions, it's just that there aren't a lot of definitive answers to the questions surrounding hep C:

"Will this work?"

"We hope so, but we don't know for sure."

"Will this make me crazy?"

"We hope not, but we don't know for sure."

"If the virus goes away, will it come back?"

"We hope not, but we can't guarantee it."

And then, even when you get a definitive answer, it leads to more questions and more nonanswers.

"How's my platelet count this month?"

"Looks good!"

Well, that's great, but it doesn't mean it'll be good the next month, or the month after that. It's just one thing after another, and it really is anxiety-producing.

We were pleased with our hep C group. Earl's virus wasn't responding but Mary's did. Problems were coming up, but people were managing and meds were adjusted and there were no big disasters. So far, so good. But I was drowning with new patients that needed help, and so I asked the group members for permission to expand. They agreed.

Our newcomers treated the established membership like landed gentry. I was happy to see how they responded in kind, proud of their hard-won expertise. The novices were full of questions about all aspects of hepatitis C. Their tendency was to look to me for the answers, but I wanted to avoid a boring lecture format. For these patients the most valuable expertise lay with experienced group members. Having already taken hepatitis C treatment, they had a credibility I lacked.

So in these question-and-answer sessions, my role was to elicit the correct answer from someone in the group rather than just giving it up myself. This is called the Socratic method of teaching; it is a wonderful way of keeping things interactive and interesting, and it keeps people from dozing off over lunch.

Let's say a new group member would ask, "Is there a cure for hepatitis C?" That was a common question. Here is an example of how the discussion might go, beginning with my question to the group in response.

DS:

What is it called when you have no detectable virus six months after the treatment is over? Who knows the answer?

GROUP MEMBER:

SVR. Sustained virologic response.

DS:

Good! What percent of people who take the treatment have an SVR?

GROUP MEMBER:

70 percent?

DS:

Okay, good guess, but that's a little high. Try again.

GROUP MEMBER:

50 percent?

DS:

That's really close. It's actually about 42 percent.

This was the statistic at the time, with standard interferon and ribavirin. Currently, with pegylated interferon and ribavirin, the number is about 55 percent.

DS:

But what does that mean for those 42 percent? Is it a cure?

GROUP MEMBER:

Probably.

DS:

Why do you say that?

GROUP MEMBER:

Because over 90 percent of people with an SVR never have virus again.

DS:

Okay, but how do you know if the SVR is a cure? Why isn't the virus hiding? We don't know for sure, do we?

Then that discussion might riff into how to decide that a cancer is cured, or how the genetics of the hepatitis C virus do not allow it to stay dormant by integrating into our own DNA, or any of a number of other topics that kept participants interested and on their toes. Believe it or not, the discussions could get that sophisticated, as established members returned over and over again and became remarkably versed in hepatitis C knowledge. Sometimes the patients in the group would just blow me away with how much they knew, and it taught me the importance of making sure the established group members didn't get bored: Their expert participation was the key to the lively interactions that were surprisingly fun, even for me. There had to be something in it for everyone, new members as well as old. That way, they would keep coming back.

Then we'd move on to another topic. "But what about side effects?" someone would ask. Those in treatment would chuckle knowingly. "Earl, what about you?" I'd say. "Let's hear from you, Phil." By the time we were done we'd put together a nice long list of awful side effects, each of which was being confronted in a positive way. That was good, the honesty about the side effects. It was constructive to bring them up.

Another thing is, you never see the doctor. In every other aspect of my life, I'm okay with the assistant. If I want to ask my agent a question, it's fine if the agent's assistant answers the question and I never talk to the agent. I don't really care. But when it came to my health, I wanted to talk to Dr. Vierling. He's a very smart guy, he's dedicated his life to this thing, and if I need answers, I want them from him. I rarely saw Dr. Vierling during my treatment. He was busy saving lives, and he had a lot of patients. There's a hepatitis epidemic in America, and John Vierling was on the front lines. But if I needed to talk to him, he was available.

Not seeing Dr. Vierling never became a problem, though, because the nurses in his office were amazing. Nurses always do the heavy lifting and, no offense to Dr. Vierling, the hepatology nurses looked a lot better to me doing it. I've always loved nurses and thanked God for them going through treatment. I get a feeling of empathy and support from them that I usually don't get from the doctor—any doctor. Dr. Vierling's head nurse, Janet Clarke, was my case manager, and she put up with a lot of nonsense from me, especially toward the end, without ever letting on what a pain in her ass I was. I was furious all the time, always screaming and yelling about something. You know: "Why do I have to take this test?" "What does this result mean?" "Why is this taking so long?" "Where the hell is Dr. Vierling?"

I was not a guy you'd be happy to see walking into your waiting room, so in that sense I wasn't a good patient. But I stuck with the protocol, which I wasn't sure I could do. Lots of people don't because it's hard, and it gets harder as time goes on.

When you come from the streets, you are no fan of authority. My new patients are wary, instinctively bonding with peers; building trust takes time. So it would be fair to say that my own patients were less concerned about seeing me, personally. They liked the importance of it, and it was good that I was around, but they were drawing more from the group experience than from me. I was also getting busier, and so around that time a physician's assistant named Barry Clements came to work at my clinic. He had a warm, natural sense of humor and a wonderful touch with the groups. I became less central to the process, even though I was usually there.

There were so many things to keep track of, with more and more patients on treatment. Fortunately there were algorithms for monitoring blood counts. At the time we would draw blood at weeks 2, 4, 8, and 12, and every four to six weeks thereafter. Interferon reduces white blood cell and platelet counts early on, starting at week 2. Sometimes the interferon dose needed to be reduced. Ribavirin, as I have already mentioned, usually causes some degree of anemia, but on occasion it can be severe. You start to see the anemia around week 4 of treatment, but by weeks 8 to 12 it has become fully manifest. I've been caught unaware by it on occasion and have let the blood count go down too low, sometimes because patients didn't show up for blood tests and sometimes because I failed to appreciate the slope of the decline.

Patients took less ribavirin if they got too anemic, and sometimes they had to stop it altogether. Nowadays a lot of us prescribe injections of erythropoietin, a hormone that stimulates the production of new red blood cells. That way most patients can stay on the full dose of ribavirin, in the hope of protecting their viral response.

Week 12 was a key time in a number of ways. A minor reason was that we checked the thyroid for the first time, because interferon has a tendency to screw it up. More important, week 12 was when we drew our first on-treatment viral load, our initial indication of whether there would be a treatment response. As we discussed earlier, the term for this test is the EVR, early virologic response. If the virus wasn't gone or hadn't declined by at least a hundredfold by then, it meant that the treatment probably wouldn't be successful. Without an EVR, there was only a 2 to 3 percent chance of an SVR. Although there was reason to believe that the liver benefited from interferon even without a viral response, that outcome was kind of a bummer anyway. My patients usually stayed on treatment regardless, because their liver disease was usually pretty advanced.

These days we do our first viral load test at week 4. The test is called the RVR, or rapid virologic response. If the virus is undetectable at that point, that indicates that your chances of responding to treatment are excellent. This particular test is sometimes used to consider shortening the duration of treatment if the results are good, or sometimes prolonging the treatment beyond six months if a sensitive genotype is not responding as rapidly as we would like.

The last key aspect of week 12 relates to depression. I'll use "depression" as a broad term for the spectrum of mood problems that interferon can cause. It actually doesn't reach its peak until week 12, but then it hangs on for the ride, chipping away at morale and perseverance. We paid extra attention to mood as the weeks went on, and asked our patients to do the same.

After the beginning of treatment, the first point on the horizon was twelve weeks in, when the viral load in my blood would be tested. If I had a lower level of HCV in my blood, that would mean the medication was working and I had achieved what Dr. Vierling called an EVR, or early virological response. I was nervous, fearing the worst, but maintained an attitude and belief that the treatment was working. I was determined to manifest an EVR. I had learned in recovery that I couldn't think myself into right action but had to act myself into right thinking. I took this approach to all the milestones in my treatment—I acted as if all of them would be positive.

I went in for the bloodwork and never looked back. When Janet called with the good news I acted as if I'd never had a doubt.

Maybe this is my imagination, but I feel as if the interferon was mostly responsible for the physical side effects, while the ribavirin took its toll mentally and emotionally.

Physically there was that terrible, flulike ache deep in the muscles. I got skin rashes. I developed floaters in my eyes, these little black specks drifting across my vision. I called Janet Clarke, panicking.

"Janet, something's wrong. I've got all these little black things floating across my eyes."

"That's why we call them floaters. Some of the patients get them." Janet had had this conversation before.

"Well, are they permanent? Are they going to go away?" I asked.

"They usually do, Chris. Sometimes they don't, but that's very rare."

JUNKIE CHRIS:

Holy shit, man! You're going blind. I knew this wasn't a good idea.

SOBER CHRIS:

We are not going blind. The floaters will go away after we complete treatment.

JUNKIE CHRIS:

She said they usually *go away. It's* rare *if they don't. You're special enough to have something rare happen to you.*

I also got canker sores, and my hair started thinning. I lost weight, which was the one aspect of the whole experience I appreciated. All of those things I attributed to the interferon. With the ribavirin, I felt it was making me fuzzy mentally. I had this constant, low-grade anxiety. I was always feeling discontented, impatient, on edge. Anything that might have been irritating before—being stuck in traffic, loud noises, somebody's odd personality tics— was ten times worse, just intolerable. I really lost any patience, any ability to tolerate frustration or irritation.

There was also a real physical component to this irritation and agitation. One of the people I reached out to was a guy who'd already gone through the treatment unsuccessfully. Later on he ended up taking an eighteen-month treatment protocol, just to make absolutely sure the HCV got wiped out. One afternoon a few months into treatment, I met him at a movie theater. About a quarter of the way through the film, I was so frazzled, so annoyed and anxious, that I had to get up and leave. I said, "I'm sorry, man, I just can't take this movie." He told me, "It's not the movie, Chris. You just can't sit still, and that's all about the medication."

It felt like all that was the impact of the ribavirin, and I hated it. My friend Bill says fifteen minutes after he swallowed the ribavirin, he could taste it—"something nasty, like it'd take the paint off your car."

One of the most profound, most frightening memories of this treatment was the feeling of hopelessness: deep, dark, and relentless, with no relief in sight. I've never felt that way before. I've never been a depressive. My outlook on life has always been seeing the glass as half full. During treatment the glass was empty and cracked. For the first six or seven months or so I was able to deal with the depression by focusing on the fact that the treatment was working and that I was saving my life, but at some point even the thought of saving my life didn't make me feel better. I never want to feel that way again, and I associate that with the ribavirin. Now, I could be completely wrong about this, but that's what it felt like to me.

That same friend who went to the movie with me said he thinks the side effects get worse over time as the medication—especially the ribavirin—builds up in your body. And since one of the side effects is a decreased ability to deal with things, well, it can become kind of a nightmare as time goes on.

We like to finger a single culprit for treatment side effects, blaming either interferon or ribavirin for one mess or another. Sometimes that's reasonable, but frequently it's not so cut-and-dried. Interferon is the one causing flu-like symptoms and reducing the white blood cell counts and platelets. Ribavirin is the primary cause of anemia. Nausea is also mostly from ribavirin, and based on the experimenting of my patients, I tell people with nausea to split up their pills (for example, one pill six times daily, or two pills three times daily, instead of three pills twice daily). Sometimes an antacid helps, or sometimes a medication that reduces nausea directly is needed.

Skin problems, including things like rashes and canker sores, happen to everyone. Hepatitis C treatment is a miracle mystery tour of dermatology. Things will crop up, move around, go away. Weird things. They itch, stick out, erupt.

Over-the-counter creams can help but may make them worse. It's good to let your doctor know about them, but don't expect to hear, "I know *exactly* what that is." You will more likely hear something like, "Yeah, that's real common. We don't know what it is, but here's something that will help." It could be a cortisone-type cream, or Benadryl, or occasionally something with antibiotics. Dry skin is very common, and here is our strategy: After you shower or bathe, take a tiny bit of petroleum jelly, rub it between your hands, then buff a very thin layer onto your dry skin. A thin layer, not a greased-pig deal. It acts kind of like plastic wrap, keeping the moisture in. If you itch, scratch with an ice cube. That has the extra benefit of numbing it up.

Interferon reduces the amount of saliva you make, and you will have a dry mouth and tend toward canker sores. Drink lots of fluid and gargle with salt water. Lemon drops or other sour candies make you salivate.

Problems with the eyes are also common and usually harmless, but we tend to worry about them more because a few serious things can happen. A lot of people get dry eyes and blurry vision because the glands secrete less moisture. But if you have eye problems, be sure to mention them to your doctor. I had a patient named Ellen who complained of blurry vision. It took nearly two months to get her an appointment with an eye doctor because there was only one who took Medicaid, but then she didn't show up. By the time we got her rescheduled, she ended up needing steroids injected directly into her eyes for a rare condition called Vogt-Koyanagi-Harada syndrome. It was caused by interferon and she went nearly blind. I wrote that case up for a medical journal, hoping to keep the same thing from happening to other people. Ellen went on to have an SVR, which was wonderful because she had cirrhosis, but at some point she started drinking again. She lost her housing and then she was found dead of a presumed drug overdose. It is hard to be female, homeless, and blind. In my mind, hepatitis C treatment will always play a role in her death.

There's nothing like a bummer of a story to circle us back to treatment-related mood disorders. This is a fact: Everyone has them. We usually think of interferon as the cause because we do know that treatment with interferon alone, such as was done early in hepatitis C, can cause depression. There are a number of reasons why ribavirin might make that worse, and certainly it does seem to add some symptoms of anxiety to the mix.

Most people seem to think that they can choose whether they will get depressed or anxious or psychotic. But you can't order up your side effects: They choose you. Of my original group of five, the one who had the worst problem with depression was Mary, who had never been diagnosed with depression in her life. She responded to the antidepressant citalopram, but not before we were treated to a few choice weeks of her mood. Many of my marginalized patients have histories of depression or something like it, often undiagnosed. They never had a doctor to make the diagnosis, after all. The general teaching is that hepatitis C treatment should be avoided in patients like these, because things could get worse. Sometimes they do. But it more often seems that patients like these—because of their lack of access to medical care—have developed compensatory strategies to deal with their illness, and they actually tolerate interferon better than the others.

The advice I give is simple: Consider an antidepressant or mood stabilizer if your mood has ever been a problem. Think about starting a low dose early, perhaps before treatment begins. That way you know you are taking something that will agree with you, and the dose can be increased if needed. Make sure you get enough sleep: Insomnia is common, and it makes all of us irritable. Take something to help with that if you need to. Benadryl is good for lot of people, but there are many other options to consider.

All those months when I was trying to find reasons not to start the protocol, I investigated alternative treatments a little bit. There were people who told me they were cured of hepatitis C by taking massive intravenous doses of vitamin C. There were folks who said laetrile and other drugs found south of the border would do the trick. I'm not a doctor, and I can't say they're wrong. But I finally decided that there's only one scientifically documented way to treat hepatitis C, and that's with interferon and ribavirin. I decided not to mess around. I was going for the most direct line from A to B, to give myself the best chance for a positive outcome. I put all my chips on the interferon-and-ribavirin protocol and said, "This is going to work." I did take vitamins and milk thistle, which I had heard strengthens the liver, and my doctor said that though there was no science to support the claim, he could say the milk thistle wouldn't do any harm.

Bill did a massive amount of research, and he took a very holistic approach. He really paid attention to his diet, he used herbal supplements, and he went to a homeopath to help him when he was trying to wean himself off the antidepressant. But he also did the same kind of hard-core interferon-and-ribavirin protocol I did. Everything else was worth doing—it made him feel better, it worked for him—but as far as I can tell, there is no real alternative to the medical treatment.

People swear by herbal medications, both for their benefits in managing the symptoms of hepatitis C as well as their help with the side effects of treatment. That's fine. Just be aware that alternative therapies have never been shown to clear the hepatitis C virus. They are also not regulated by the FDA, so use caution with outsize claims—a few herbs, such as kava, can cause liver failure—and beware of your wallet. If you are going to use alternative therapies, be sure to consult a qualified practitioner, and let your doctor know that you are taking them—it's not something we always remember to ask about.

One thing that did help me a great deal was yoga. I did a very strenuous yoga practice an hour and a half every day I was in treatment. It was a vinyasa flow class not far from where I lived, consisting of about fifty minutes of continual movement through various standing yoga postures followed by forty minutes of inversions, back bends, and stretching. It's a difficult practice when I'm healthy, and sometimes I'd have to leave early because I was so weak from the medication. But I was there every day, and that helped with my mood and with the body aches by opening me up and releasing all those endorphins. Bill did the same thing, and the way he put it was, "Whenever I did yoga, I felt normal for a couple of hours afterward. It's like my body forgot about everything else that was going on."

Since 1992 I've maintained a practice of daily meditation and weekly chanting at an ashram in West Los Angeles. My practice suffered during my eleven months of treatment, because it was difficult for me to sit still. But I kept attending, and when I was able to meditate, my mood and the way I felt physically improved. There is a spiritual axiom that if there is pain or discomfort, the solution is to dive deeper into it instead of trying to avoid it. This is not easy to do, but my experience has shown me that it works.

Exercise is the last thing you'll feel like doing, but it is one thing you should commit to. It really does help; maybe it is the endorphins, who knows? You don't have to do a heavy workout every day, just do something, a little bit, even if you don't want to. Even a walk around the block will help you feel better. Every day get out and just do a little something.

I also found that drinking lots and lots of water helped. I mean, a gallon a day, something like that. For one thing it's always a good idea to stay hydrated. More important, I thought of it as flushing my body out, washing away the bad effects of the medications.

That's worth repeating: Drink lots of water, fifteen to twenty eight-ounce glasses a day. About a gallon, as Chris said. Water is the number one thing to help with that unpleasant, headachy, viral way you will feel. We don't know why it works, but every single person I have had on treatment swears by it. That is a lot of water to drink, so keep a bottle with you and sip it all the time.

I had one patient named Tom who drank too much water, something like two or three gallons a day, but we weren't completely sure. He was just trying to be an extra-good patient. In the process he washed the sodium from his body, and that gave him a seizure and a trip to the hospital. I learned to explain my water enthusiasm a little more specifically.

A gallon a day is enough. Oh, and try to finish it up in the early evening. Otherwise you'll be up all night.

The thing that was hardest to deal with was the way my sleep was disrupted. I didn't get a good night's sleep for eleven months, and that takes an incredible toll on you. It affects your health, it impacts your moods, it affects how well you deal with things generally.

Like I said earlier, I'm very wary about taking any kind of mind-altering drug. I've had major mouth surgeries and back issues where doctors had said, "You should take something," and I never did. Not because I'm brave or tough, but because I'm terrified of waking up that narcotic craving again, the eight-hundred-pound gorilla. But eventually, I had to start taking something just to get some sleep. I took Tylenol PM, which worked. If I had to travel or was really having a hard time sleeping, I'd take Ambien because I'd been told it's one of the least addictive, least dangerous drugs of that kind. Still, I tried to keep the Ambien to a minimum.

Insomnia is common. It is probably mostly from interferon, along the lines of the way you sleep poorly when you're sick with the flu. Get the insomnia under control, or it will wear you down big-time. Confine caffeine to the first part of the day. Take naps, but keep them brief if you are staying up all night. Benadryl (the generic form, diphenhydramine, is one of the ingredients in Tylenol PM) can help with sleep and may be worth a try. If that doesn't work, then ask your doctor for something else.

Many of my patients with insomnia also have a history of depression or a related disorder. A good number of antidepressants and mood stabilizers cause drowsiness as a side effect, and this is a great time to help both with one pill. Plus at my clinic we try to stay away from controlled substances to the extent that we can. Some of the things we use in this way are amitriptyline, trazodone, mirtazapine, or quetiapine, but there are many others. Regular sleeping pills like Ambien are perfectly fine and sometimes necessary. Just try not to use them every single night because your body will become accustomed to them.

On a different note, some antidepressants have the contrary effect: They tend to keep you awake. We have talked a lot about insomnia, but sometimes the problem is the opposite: sleeping all day, every day. I'll try one of these stimulating kinds of antidepressants, like bupropion or venlafaxine, when my patients can't stay awake or have no energy whatsoever. They usually help to some extent.

Whatever I was taking, I kept in touch with Dr. Vierling and the nurses about it as well as with the friends I rely on to stay clean and sober. I learned early on in my recovery that I am only as sick as my secrets, so I didn't keep any from the people who keep me honest in recovery. So many over-the-counter drugs can build up in your liver, so you have to make sure you don't overdo it. Dr. Vierling had me switch from Tylenol to Advil and back. Every once in a while I'd take Aleve or Motrin for the muscle aches, and Dr. Vierling had me switch those around too.

Muscle and joint aches are a problem for everyone on hepatitis C treatment. It is generally fine to take things like acetaminophen and ibuprofen (also known by the brand names Tylenol and Advil) or one of the other over-the-counter painkillers for your aches and pains. You will definitely have them. But Chris is right: Check with your doctor just to be safe.

Like I said earlier, my motto is, You can't hit a moving target. When I'm stressed, I go for motion and activity and drama and distraction. The whole time I was on the protocol, I was very stressed and very distracted. There was all the drama with Carrie, arguing and breaking up and getting back together. There was the ongoing battle with my ex-wife, and trying to maintain some kind of relationship with my kids. There was my work with *Extra*, which was ridiculous and not really working out. I was back to pretty much living in my car, with my toilet kit and my yoga clothes and my suit. I was always driving between my kids' house, my cousin Maria's house where the mouse and I lived, Carrie's house in Hollywood, and *Extra*. I was constantly in motion. I never sat still long enough to feel my feelings. I'd drive and I'd listen to really loud music, while ranting and raving on the telephone.

I didn't plan it that way, and I can't recommend the strategy to anyone else, but looking back on it, I think all this drama and distraction helped me get through the fear as well as the physical and mental challenges of those eleven months. If I had cleared out everything else in my life so that the treatment was the only thing I was paying attention to, I might have sunk down into a place where I wouldn't have been able to continue.

My patients are experts at creating drama and bringing it into their lives. Sometimes they manage to bring it to the clinic as well. I suspect this kind of drama is different from what Chris is suggesting: Ours tends to involve blue uniforms and flashing lights. It plays better on the screen or the stage.

That said, I know what he means. Distractions help pass the time. Our hepatitis C group is one such distraction, and that is a part of its plan. A mandate to get up out of bed. To shower and dress. To learn something new. To help someone else, knowing that you need it more.

But if there is something major coming up, like a big trip or exams or something like that, treatment should probably begin afterward. "Get your ducks in a row before you start," is what we say. Though no fault of your own, there may be regrets if you start too soon. One of my patients went to court on a minor traffic infraction and flipped off the judge: His fine went up, way up. Another took on his younger cousin at a family reunion, over some incident involving a garden hose that had taken place thirty-two years earlier. His cousin, who now had him by six inches and something like seventy pounds, blackened his eye and took out his left front tooth.

Distractions yes, drama no.

While I was getting ready to start treatment, I was filled with dread and fear of the unknown, only to find the reality wasn't nearly as bad as I'd thought it might be. This was a huge relief and I lived off that feeling for a while. That, coupled with the never-ending drama of my life, kept me from slipping into the black hole of hep C treatment that I always imagined might be waiting for me. But a few months in, the whole thing really started getting to me. I felt like I was in quicksand, and the harder I tried to keep it together, the deeper I sank. For months I felt like I was managing my treatment and then suddenly the treatment was managing me in a very scary way. It got harder and harder to ignore the fact I was waking up every day feeling hopeless and depressed.

I reached a point where I had to talk myself through it every time I took the medication.

SOBER CHRIS:
Okay, Chris, now you're going take the interferon. You'll feel okay for twenty-four hours, then the flu will visit for a while, then you'll feel better.

JUNKIE CHRIS:
Don't forget those nasty little pills that make you feel like you want to swan-dive off the Hollywood sign.

Continuation

SOBER CHRIS:

It's not me, it's the drugs.

JUNKIE CHRIS:

What's the difference? You still feel like shit!

SOBER CHRIS:

There's a big difference. When I'm done with the treatment, I'll be me again.

Treatment does not get easier as time goes on. Most people don't know that the number of treatment discontinuations in the second half of treatment is just about the same as in the first half. Everyone is worried about those first few weeks, when the flulike symptoms are at their worst. The thing is, you are prepared for that. It is harder to prepare for the remaining weeks of permanent, achy fatigue, irritability, brain fog, and the rest. You will get tired of being tired. Your mood will worsen, the symptoms will accumulate. You will have pissed off most of your friends and family members. Don't let down your guard: There is no time during treatment that the challenge is over until you finish that very last dose.

One of the issues that people always worry about is, How is this treatment going to affect my work? Will I be able to work every day? The way I was making a living was piecemeal and precarious, which caused its own anxiety, but the advantage was it allowed me some control over when I worked. I didn't have to show up and work eight or ten hours every single day—including the day after I'd had my interferon shot, when I felt at my worst.

I have no recollection of getting any acting jobs the year I was in treatment for hep C, but according to the Internet Movie Database, I did a movie called *Hitters* that came out in 2002, which meant it was probably shot during 2001. I don't remember anything about it—the set, the other actors in it, nothing. I haven't seen it to this day.

I know I never went off on anyone at *Extra*, although I remember getting increasingly annoyed with the celebrities I interviewed. I was putting together segments on everything from actors against the war in Afghanistan to Arnold Schwarzenegger's possible run for governor. I became more and more resentful about being the interviewer and not the interviewee, and the fact I felt lousy while I had to act hyper-interested and bubbly about whatever it was the celebrity was selling only made it worse. I didn't tell anyone at *Extra* that I was being treated for hep C. I was worried they'd fire me, and I couldn't afford to get fired.

My friend Bill handled this very differently. He's an actor too, and also a real estate agent with several long-term clients, and he cut way back on his real estate work while he was being treated. However, he did do a couple of deals, including one with a client he knew well and some of the client's family members. We'll call the client Stan. They were all in Bill's office talking about the deal and . . . well, I'll let Bill tell it.

It was a $500,000 house that ultimately became worth about $1.2 million. They were squeezing the seller for a thousand dollars and I just went off on *them.* "*You guys are totally unreasonable, I can't believe you're doing this,*" *on and on. They were kind of shocked, and they left.*

I remember sitting in my office and thinking, I would never have done that if I wasn't taking this crap. I would have made pretty much the same point, but I would have said it differently, with different language, different inflection and tone. So I called up Stan and I apologized, and he said, "It's that fucking medicine you're taking."

I said, "Yeah, I know it is. I'm sorry."

"*Don't worry about it.*"

I was very open about being on interferon, almost to a fault. But in this case, I think it was good that Stan knew up front what was going on, and I didn't have to explain everything after I'd already gone off on him.

So the question of whether and how to disclose your treatment status at your workplace isn't one that has black-and-white answers. Bill and I made different decisions based on our individual circumstances, and those decisions worked out okay for each of us. I think the key is in *consciously* making those decisions—and being willing to reconsider your decisions as needed.

Another friend who's been treated for HCV—the one who went to the movies with me—owns his own company. At first he tried to keep up with the business and just cut his hours back a little. But one day he realized that he couldn't do it anymore: "I was yelling at everyone, out of control, and in terms of my concentration and focus, I was only operating at about 30 or 40 percent. I thought, 'I've got to excuse myself from this.' And I did. I turned over the company to somebody else until I was done."

This guy was determined to maintain his workload but his commitment to beating the disease was his first priority. He was in treatment for the second time and he was on a very difficult eighteen-month protocol. He couldn't keep working and finish treatment, so he had to revise his original plans and step away from the job. He made it through and he's cured today.

Many people continue working to some extent, but some can't. It really just depends. Things like concentration and memory will be shot, so if you do something like accounting for a living, work may be impossible. People who do dangerous work like crane operators or who work on highrises need to be put on desk jobs or go out on disability. A patient of mine named Marvin crashed his forklift a couple of times before he told his surprisingly understanding boss about the treatment. Last, remember the irritability. If being pleasant and cheerful needs to be part of your job, watch out.

I know people who've undergone both chemotherapy and interferon treatment, and some have said the interferon was tougher. I don't know personally, and I hope never to find out, but I know one of the problems I ran into was that you often don't look anywhere near as bad on interferon as you feel. As time goes on the people in your support system can start losing patience with you because they don't have the steady sick-person visual. I remember Carrie threw a big party at her house a few months into my treatment. On the night of the party I was so exhausted I went to bed at eleven o'clock, long before the party was over. The next day she was furious. "How could you do that to me on my birthday?" Well, I could do it because I wasn't physically capable of doing anything else. She didn't understand that, really, and because I didn't look or act sick, she forgot that I was. Partly her reaction was about her and about our relationship, but it was also about the fact that the effects of treatment were not always readily apparent. I still had most of my hair and all of my limbs, my skin wasn't flaking off or peeling away, I wasn't bleeding from the ears or anything like that. I looked tired. I didn't look like a dead man walking, which is how I felt.

Many people on hepatitis C treatment seem to look better than they feel. But that is not always the best of circumstances, particularly on those days when you are feeling particularly annoyed or having homicidal fantasies. Ask any family member and you will see what I mean.

One good part about that (Ladies, pay attention!) is that you are not going to go bald. You hair will thin, and you will experience some of the anxiety men go through when their hairline begins receding, like checking the shower and sink drains in despair. Your hair can also get kind of dry and cracked looking, and you may want to consider a shorter cut. A wonderful patient of mine named Mark, who set records for belligerence and the use of foul language in our groups, had straight black hair and it came to stand untamably on end. That enraged him. He was actually enraged about his hair. No amount of gel would smooth it down, and he complained bitterly about looking like a "fucking porcupine," a circumstance that gradually dissipated after the treatment was over. On the other hand, some of my African American patients have been very pleased with the effects of interferon, because their hair straightened out for a time.

Aside from this, though, the truth is that not everyone looks great on hepatitis C treatment. Some people's dispositions are not that sturdy, and they look sallow, gray, and sick. They feel that way, and probably they get more sympathy, deservedly so. But many others look quite fine. I may be able to tell the difference because I know them well, but other people can't.

I kept trying to maintain a relationship with my kids because I swore I wouldn't do to them what my father did to my sisters and me, which was disappear once he and my mother split up. I kept trying to make the massive, falling-down house I was squatting in into a home where they'd feel comfortable, and it wasn't working. My kids and I had always lived in little places, almost like hobbit houses, and their mom was great about cooking good food and making everything warm and cozy. The house I was living in was huge, drafty, and dirty. Add to that my deficiencies in the homemaking skills department, and you have three miserable kids. One Sunday I tried to make pizza for us, and it burned because the oven was broken. They'd come over and swim or play tennis, but they couldn't stand the house and never wanted to spend the night there. They were also furious at me for leaving their mother and wrecking their family, which didn't help in my efforts to have them spend more time with me.

I would get frustrated and my patience was being severely stretched by the medication. It was a challenging time, trying to weather this divorce with significantly depleted resources. I needed to be better than my usual self, and I couldn't even *get* to my usual self. To be honest, looking back, I'm not sure anything would have been different if I hadn't been sick. I might have been less distracted and more committed to doing whatever I needed to do to make sure my children were comfortable in my life. But I was being medicated in a way that made me physically sick and mentally depressed, and I was in crisis. Still, I kept trying.

When Thanksgiving came around, I wanted a nice, Norman Rockwell–style dinner with them. Bill came over, and I wasn't going to risk another pizza incident, so we ordered food from a grocery store near my house. I laid out this fancy Thanksgiving dinner and my kids hated it. I could see it on their faces. They hated the meal because it had all sorts of nuts and spices in the stuffing and gravy—not at all like what their mom made. They didn't want to be at my cold, dirty house for Thanksgiving, eating a gourmet turkey dinner. They wanted to be at their house eating the dinner they were used to, and they wanted me to be there too. They tried, but there was no way for them to be thankful or happy.

It was in that moment that I realized my kids weren't

going be a part of my life in the way I imagined, not at that point. It was so upsetting, so deflating. It was like a big balloon with the air leaking out of it—that terrible Thanksgiving dinner.

This gets us back to the irritability and drama issues; we've already discussed these in detail. That is one reason why we try to get people to discuss their hepatitis C treatment with family. It is not always easy to discuss these things. But its importance is that you could behave in ways that you won't want to remember, and there are bridges you don't want to burn. It will take others to put out the flames.

Chris's misery at Thanksgiving is one such example. He was miserable, and it was contagious. That was interferon doing its thing.

Not long after, almost eight months in, I hit some kind of wall and I knew there was no way over, under, or around it. I fought it for a few days and then I did something I swore I would never do. It was another beautiful California day. I was in the teardown, in the middle of the day, all alone. Even the mouse was gone. I lay on my bed in total defeat. The only thought in my mind was, "I can't do this anymore." In that moment I gave up.

I've never been a hopeless person. I can always see a ray of light somewhere, always, no matter what. I was brought up that way and it's part of my nature, but the treatment obliterated that. I was in a black hole and I couldn't see any light, any way out, anywhere. I was thinking about suicide and I decided, "I have to ask Dr.

Vierling for antidepressants." As soon as I made that decision, I felt a little hope. Being a drug addict, I have great
confidence that pills can alleviate whatever condition I
have. I thought, Okay, I just have to make it through one
more night. Tomorrow I'm going to take this pill and I'll
feel better.

The next day, when I went to Dr. Vierling's office, he
said, "Look, Chris, it takes weeks for the antidepressant
to be effective. By then you'll be close to the end of treatment, and you'll have to wean yourself off the antidepressant."

JUNKIE CHRIS:
Well, screw that! I want an instant feel-better fix!

SOBER CHRIS:
There's no such thing. Looks like it's gut-check time.

JUNKIE CHRIS:
Looks like it's quitting time!

SOBER CHRIS:
*You really want to risk not getting the one sneaky hep
C bug hiding deep down inside somewhere?*

JUNKIE CHRIS:
We got them all, man.

SOBER CHRIS:
If we quit because of you and the hep C comes back, I

won't forgive you until the day you die—which you're
gonna wish comes sooner rather than later.

There was a half measure, though, and I took it. Dr.
Vierling suggested I cut back on my interferon and ribavirin levels. He reasoned that I'd had an EVR early on and
that a drop in dosage wouldn't be detrimental to my treatment. I felt a little like I was quitting, but I did it anyway
and felt better, which renewed my commitment to finish
the protocol.

As you have gathered, I am a fan of antidepressants and
mood stabilizers. But I am also a fan of nausea medications, skin creams, antacids, sleeping pills: anything that
helps—whatever it takes to get through treatment. Mental
side effects are a big deal for some people and can be cumu-
lative. They can be dangerous and lead to treatment discontinuations. But medications can help. They are not mental
handcuffs. They just let you function while you finish the
treatment.

I looked at the data from one of our first studies to see
how many of our patients used psychiatric medications during hepatitis C treatment. About 40 percent were taking
something at the start, and 86 percent were using something
by the time treatment was over. The remaining 14 percent
made *me* want to take something, if I recall correctly. But
here is the good news: We had been told that our patients
couldn't be treated. They were too sick, or crazy, or unstable.
But they did quite fine. Their outcomes were similar to everyone else's.

Chapter 7

Completion

I remember the last shot of interferon. Carrie was out of town and she'd asked me to call her so she could be a part of it. I called but she didn't answer her phone, which pissed me off so I did the shot on my own, knowing it would make her angry. I kid you not—I was really passive-aggressive while I was going through treatment. The mouse was there and it seemed fitting that I end my long road of treatment with my furry friend. Carrie called at two o'clock in the morning and I told her I'd already done the shot. She got mad and hung up on me.

It was a relief to be done. I remember being amazed and proud of myself that I'd gotten through it—without a whole lot of grace, but I'd done it. I'd kept all five of my intentions. But the relief was short-lived. I was concerned about two things: The hepatitis C might come back, and I was going to get fat. With both those things, it takes time to find out. It takes months for your body to return to anything that feels like normal. And you have to wait six months and get another test to find out if everything you went through really worked and the virus is, once and for all, out of your body for good.

Six months after I put that last syringe loaded with interferon into my left thigh I walked into Cedars-Sinai for the test I'd been thinking about for the past year and a half—the test that would tell me if I was one of the lucky ones who had achieved an SVR. I careened between nervousness, denial, and trying to stay positive.

JUNKIE CHRIS:

What if it's come back, man?

SOBER CHRIS:

We gave it our best shot. It's out of our hands now.

JUNKIE CHRIS:

You shouldn't have cut back at the end! What if you missed one of the little bastards?

SOBER CHRIS:

Be cool, my junkie alter ego. Let's wait and see what the doctor has to say.

At some point in the next couple of weeks Dr. Vierling called to say he had good news—the virus was gone. There was no detectable hepatitis C virus in my body.

Completion

After one of my patients took his last dose, he got a brick and bashed his final syringe and ribavirin bottle into tiny little pieces. He had been fantasizing about this for months. The problem was, he told me, he got so exhausted from doing it that he had to spend the rest of the day in bed. You can't win with this stuff.

The countdown becomes an obsession. But for most of my patients, as it was for Chris, taking that last dose is more of a letdown. You take it, then nothing. It's just over. You still feel just as crappy as you did yesterday, plus you come to realize that there is nothing more you can do beyond this point to help kill the virus. It is either gone or it isn't.

That is a long time to wait, six months, to find out if the treatment was successful. You do not suddenly feel better the week after the treatment is over either. First of all these are long-acting medications, and they linger for a period of several weeks. Blood counts begin improving soon thereafter, but the rest takes some time. Rashes slowly fade. Your hair will seemingly take forever to regrow, as that is its nature. The fatigue and irritability also lift slowly, usually over a period of months. That never happens fast enough: I have had patients say it took one or two years. On average it takes three to six months.

We have discussed what the SVR means, the sustained virologic response. It is a definition. Your blood is drawn six months after you finish treatment. If there is no detectable virus, then you have had an SVR. Congratulations, the treatment worked. About 55 percent of people who take the treatment get this news. We tell them that they are probably cured.

There is some controversy about the word *cure*. A couple of research groups have found genetic material from hepatitis C in the body's immune cells and liver, long after the virus has gone. They cite this as evidence that hepatitis C is incurable.

On the other hand most of us use the word *cure* for practical reasons based on clinical data. One recent study by Dr. Mark Swain and his colleagues in Canada showed that, of 997 people with an SVR, only 8 of them ever had recurrent virus, even after lengthy follow-up. That is less than a 1 percent chance of ever seeing it again. Plus hepatitis C can't integrate into your DNA because its genetic material is RNA. Without the enzyme reverse transcriptase, the key to HIV's resilience, hepatitis C just can't get in. Last, when you have an SVR, your liver repairs itself and you can no longer transmit the virus to anyone. For all practical purposes it is gone. So I'm okay with the word *cure* here.

Not everyone is as fortunate as I was when confronting hepatitis C. I was diagnosed before it was too late. I had the easiest genotype to treat—a genotype that is relatively uncommon in North America. I had access to the drugs that saved my life, and I had excellent medical care. I had a built-in support group in recovery that sustained me, keeping me going when I didn't think I could. Most people in this country and in the world are not so lucky. This is a terrible, tricky disease, and depending on the specific genotype, the response rate can be 50 percent or less. Researchers are also discovering that different patient populations have different response rates. Among African Americans, it can be more like 40 percent.

Completion

Whether or not you will respond depends on a number of things. Many of them you cannot change. We have previously discussed that fact that, overall, about 55 percent of people treated for hepatitis C clear it or achieve an SVR. The main factor that determines the probability that this will happen is your genotype, the strain of hepatitis C that you started with.

The majority of people in the United States, something like 75 percent, have genotype 1. Unfortunately that is the hardest one to get rid of—it is more resistant to the medications that we are using today. If you have this genotype, then you are usually treated for forty-eight weeks and have to take a full dose of ribavirin, typically 1,000 to 1,200 mg daily, usually five or six pills. The studies suggest that your chance of an SVR is about 40 to 45 percent or so, a little less than a coin toss.

For the lucky minority who have genotypes 2 or 3, the so-called good genotypes, the picture is rosier. Twenty-four weeks is the typical duration of treatment, and the ribavirin dose is usually more like 800 mg, or four pills, per day. SVR rates are much better, on the order of 85 percent. That is a pretty good number. Genotype 2, the one Chris had, is the most sensitive of all. Genotype 3 can be a little more tenacious, and nowadays sometimes we end up treating it for forty-eight weeks, just to be sure. Genotype 4 resembles genotype 1 in its response rates, and although we know less about genotypes 5 and 6, they are probably somewhere in between.

There are other things that can affect treatment outcomes. One that Chris mentioned is race: African Americans have lower response rates than Caucasians. Some of this is because

African Americans are more likely to have genotype 1, on the order of 90 percent, which makes it harder to clear. But even when matched for genotype, outcomes for African Americans are modestly lower. That appears to relate to genetic differences in the immune response: The baseline response is lower in African Americans, and we don't exactly know why. Interferon works by boosting the immune response, but when the baseline starts lower, the boost is not sufficient to clear virus in as many people. And so outcomes are less successful: SVR rates are about 40 percent overall in African Americans, as compared with 55 percent in large-scale studies in which African Americans represent a minority.

This has an interesting correlate. You may remember that the liver damage from hepatitis C is not the virus's fault. It is the immune system's drive to expel it that wreaks havoc. But since African Americans have a less aggressive response on the whole, they are also less likely than Caucasians to have an inflamed liver, and therefore are less likely to develop advanced liver disease. It is a double-edged sword.

As to outcomes in Latinos, it appears that they are somewhere in between. There is little published data on hepatitis C outcomes in Asians. But one study that I saw suggested that they had the best response rates of all.

Coinfection with HIV is another issue. Hepatitis C causes liver scarring about four times faster if you have HIV, and treatment outcomes are modestly lower. There is some evidence that outcomes decline further as HIV advances. For this reason, and because we do know that hepatitis C treatment is less successful with advanced liver disease, HIV coinfection is one situation that leads me to be more aggressive with treatment. I am far more inclined to suggest hepatitis C treatment if you also have HIV.

Another factor predicting outcomes in a small way, as just mentioned, is the amount of liver scarring. For instance, treatment is less successful if you have cirrhosis, and the less scarring, the better. Some doctors respond to this by treating pretty much everyone, figuring that success rates will only decline over time. That is not unreasonable, but I happen to be a little more conservative. A big part of that is my patient population, but I also know that the damage progresses slowly, and I am hopeful that we'll have some new medications, and better treatment outcomes, in a few years.

That said, when a person has something called acute hepatitis C, which means that the viral infection has been present for six months or less, treatment outcomes are wonderful. More than 90 percent of people with acute hepatitis C can expect an SVR, even with the more challenging genotypes and even with a foreshortened treatment course. This is one circumstance where I will suggest treatment regardless of the amount of liver damage. Outcomes are just that good.

There are a few other factors predicting outcomes. People with a high viral load have more virus in their bodies, and so it is a little harder to clear. Thin people respond better than overweight people. Females have better outcomes than males: These factors are probably related, as women tend to be smaller. Young people respond better than older people. There are things like too much fat in the liver, or too much iron, which reduce outcomes. That is why you shouldn't take iron supplements without checking first with your doctor. You should only take iron if you need it.

We talk a lot about predicting outcomes, but the ones mentioned so far are difficult, if not impossible, to change. But there is one thing you can do to help with success: Take all your medications, all the time, on time. The data is clear on this. If you take at least 80 percent of your medications for at least 80 percent of the projected duration of treatment, you will be in the highest outcome category. That seems obvious, but the medications will play tricks on you. There will be days when you will not feel well. You want to get up and around. You skip a dose and feel better. On another day you do the same, and so forth. Your virus might even appear to be undetectable through all this, but remember that it can still be lurking in your liver. If you give it a chance to hide, it will. Take all your medications. Work with your doctor to make that happen.

Which brings up yet another thing—paying for your treatment. It can be a problem even if you have insurance, and many people don't. Over the last few years, as I've traveled around and talked about this disease, I've heard heartbreaking stories about being denied coverage, or people losing their jobs while they're being treated for hep C, and they ask me questions like "Should I go on disability?" "How much of my treatment will be covered by my insurance?" "Can my employer fire me if I have to take time off?"

Those are complicated questions that vary widely from one individual to another. I could try to cobble together a few paragraphs about HMOs and POSs but I'm not an expert, and it'd be too easy to tell you something inaccurate or misleading. Fortunately there are some amazing resources available online, offering free, detailed, specific guidance, and we've pulled together a few of them to include at the back of the book.

I believe that the primary tool of the insurance companies is a magic eight ball. Remember those, with fluid and the miracle jewel inside, that would answer your question? You try to get a medication covered. Somebody at the insurance company shakes the ball and turns it over. An answer comes up in the window; "Coverage denied." "Pre-existing condition." "Nonformulary medication." "Procedure not indicated." "Sorry, try again." They record the decision and send it back. That's how they decide. I really believe that.

For those out there who have been treated unsuccessfully there still is hope. They can be treated again. Often doctors recommend a longer protocol the second time around. And the drugs are being refined all the time. Look at how HIV treatment has developed, with more specialized and better-targeted drug cocktails. HCV treatment is moving in the same direction—although progress would be a lot faster if there were more money and more public pressure directed that way.

There is good news about hepatitis C treatment: It is successful more than half the time. It is almost miraculous that this has all taken place in a period of two decades. But then there is a sizable minority that don't respond, something like 45 percent. After all you put into the treatment, that news can be devastating.

My patient Johnny did everything right. He had come

from the streets, using heroin, cocaine, and alcohol. He stopped those and began taking an antidepressant. We started his treatment, and he took every dose. He had no detectable virus through the entire treatment course. Six months after he finished, the virus returned. There were reasons for this: He was African American, he had genotype 1, he had advanced liver disease, and he was older and male. Those all weighed against him. But just the same he was distraught. He had a major relapse to crack cocaine, and disappeared for well over a year.

But now Johnny is back. I am glad of that, because we have more in our tool kit. There is retreatment. There is longer treatment. There is another interferon, called consensus interferon, which can help.

And then there are new medications: There are a host of them in the pipeline. There are protease inhibitors, polymerase inhibitors, longer-acting interferons, and the list goes on and on. It is reasonable to expect some to hit the market in the next few years, but don't expect a miracle—hepatitis C is a lot trickier than you'd think.

Remember how you make more than a trillion new hepatitis C virus particles every day? On average, each of those new virus particles harbors one genetic mutation, hepatitis C's brilliant mechanism for evading the immune response. But that will also become its mechanism for developing resistance to some of these new medications. We don't see resistance to interferon and ribavirin even with stops and starts in treatment and poor compliance because the drugs work like cluster bombs, collectively attacking the virus in many different ways. But most of the new hepatitis C medications are more like laser beams, and each day the virus has one trillion new opportunities to create the perfect resistance shield. And resistance is exactly what we see. It develops very quickly when these new, highly specific medications are taken alone: The virus declines dramatically over the first several days, but soon thereafter new, resistant virus populations are already detected in the blood.

That doesn't mean these new medications won't be any good. It simply means that we will need to combine them with interferon, and probably also ribavirin, for the foreseeable future. Using that kind of combination protocol, we are expecting substantial improvements in treatment outcomes with shorter durations of therapy. We would like to have a miracle drug but there isn't one on the horizon. Hepatitis C is just too tricky. But it is still a very exciting time, and there is much reason for hope.

I know my treatment for hepatitis C happened at the exact moment in my life it was supposed to happen. I knew it was going to be a transformative experience. I said that at the very beginning. It was time for me to go into the depths of myself, and I made a conscious choice that I was going to come back up a different person. I went into this illness with that in mind and that was what sustained me. A lot of things came together at that point in my life, and the urgency created by the fact that I might die made that period revolutionary. I'm a different person than I was then, closer to my true self. Part of that came from the possibility of my life ending, right then. I've died many, many times during my addiction, but I've never been confronted with the possibility of really dying in sobriety. At that point in my life, everything came together in a way that enabled me to do what I needed to do. I look at that as a big turning point in my existence.

Until I was thirty-one, I had what I call junkie manhole emotional capability. I had developed this in my youth as a defense to the trauma of my parents' divorce and the assassinations of my two uncles, and nurtured it through my addiction to drugs for seventeen years. I could actually make it so that nothing mattered and no one could hurt me. That's how shut down I was. Recovery has been a long process of opening up. All the stuff that I'd buried for years in the manhole begin surfacing, and the more things surface, the more you realize is down there. The surfacing and the bubbling up had already led to a lot of changes in my life, a lot of upheaval. After I started the hep C protocol, the anger started kicking in, and as I've found throughout my recovery, everything that happens in my life has a perfect purpose.

One day I was in that dingy, drafty house, pacing back and forth, trying to figure out what to do next so I wouldn't have to deal with the facts that my life was falling apart, I had a life-threatening illness, and I had just embarked on this course of treatment that was going to make me really miserable and sick for eleven months.

The phone rang, and it was a writer who wanted to interview me for yet another book about the Kennedys. He had previously written *The Kennedy Women* and now he wanted to know what it was like to be a Kennedy man.

Please! I was angry already and that call infuriated me. I told him I wasn't in the mood to discuss it and to write me a letter explaining why I should talk to him, and I hung up. He wrote a note relaying a story about one of my cousins doing something he thought was heroic and arguing that the world needed to know this story. I called him to tell him I'd never heard the story, didn't think it was particularly heroic, and that if the world needed to know the story my cousin should tell it. I slammed the phone down, but as soon as the receiver hit the cradle I had an inspiration: I'm writing my own book. I didn't particularly think I had much of a story to tell, but I was angry enough to try. Besides, I could die, and that seemed like a decent enough reason to try. And the worst-case scenario was that my kids would have a book by their father telling them who he was.

I didn't know if I could write a book or if anyone would care enough to read it—I just started to write. Instead of letting somebody else appropriate my life and tell my story, I decided to tell my story my way. I wrote like my life depended on it, and when it looked like somebody might actually publish it, I realized I'd have to go out and sell the book.

Right around that time I got a phone call from a treatment center in Indianapolis, asking me to come there and talk about addiction and recovery at their annual fundraiser. I said yes, not because I wanted to be an advocate for recovery, hep C, or anything else, but because I figured I could use the experience. I was going to have to promote my book, and much of the book was about recovering from addiction. It was not a subject I had spent a lot of time talking about publicly outside of groups of people in recovery. At that point hepatitis C was not really a big part of my story. I gave it half a page in my memoir, *Symptoms of Withdrawal.*

When I got to Indianapolis I was scheduled to do some press events, and at the first interview a reporter stuck a microphone in my face and said, "What's it like being a heroin addict, Chris?" Not the type of question you want to be asked in front of a television camera. I fell back on my political acumen—that is, using words to get out of tight spots. I got through it, but I knew I had made a terrible mistake opening my mouth, and I was even beginning to think I shouldn't do the book. Just go home, keep my mouth shut, and be a good boy. But I had another interview to do, this one on the radio. The station had a window facing the street, kind of like the *Today* show, but instead of Matt Lauer there were two guys who just wanted dish on sex, drugs, and Marilyn Monroe. They're asking these questions, and I'm just thinking how much I don't want to be there, looking out the big picture window onto Monument Circle on a very cold winter day in Indianapolis—and then this homeless guy walks up to the window. He holds up a sign that reads, "Can you help me get sober?" His name was Lawrence, he was fifty years old, he'd been living in a Dumpster for five years, and he was the person I went there to talk to—although I hadn't known it until that moment. I haven't shut up since.

That night at the benefit I met a woman named Joyce, who was one of the cochairs of the event, and she told me that she would read my book when it came out. A year and a half later I got a call from Joyce as she was driving from Chicago back to Indianapolis. She said, "I told you I'd read your book, and I have. I didn't know you had hepatitis C. Did you know I work for Roche? We make the interferon you took."

JUNKIE CHRIS:
They also make Valium, and we took a lot of that, remember?

"No kidding?" I said to Joyce, ignoring Junkie Chris.

"Yeah, I work in government relations. I bet you didn't know the enormity of the public health crisis involving hepatitis C."

"All I know is that I had it, and now I don't."

"Well, would you like to find out?"

"Sure!"

So she started telling me about the health crisis I'd been a part of, a crisis I didn't have any idea existed. She said, "Are you aware that there are four times the number of people with HCV than have HIV? And when people are coinfected with both, they're more likely to die of HCV?" She told me that she wanted me to work with them on a new public education campaign called Hep C STAT!, which stands for Stop, Test, And Treat. The idea was to get people who have been exposed to the risk factors for hepatitis C to get tested. I checked out the program and the people involved. It looked good, so I said yes.

Never in a million years did I think that I'd be working with a drug company to promote awareness about an illness I was cured of by a drug manufactured by that company. And yet that's exactly what happened.

It's come full circle. The drug that made me angry enough and crazy enough to write my own memoir led me to work with the company that makes the drug that saved my life. I had no intention of becoming an advocate for hep C awareness. I mean, how many people diagnosed with a disease end up doing that? But when there's a need and there's an opportunity and it fits, then it makes sense. And I do believe it all happened because everything fell into place at the right time. What if that guy had called me while I was just la-di-da-ing through my life and I wasn't panicked about the possibility of dying and completely angry? I might have just talked to him and he'd have said thanks and gone off and written his book and I'd never have written mine.

Our hepatitis C group became popular. Unfortunately not everyone had been successful. Of the original group, Mary and Linette had SVRs. Cinnamon's virus came back after treatment, but pegylated interferon did the trick a few years later. Phil wasn't responding, and he got discouraged and eventually stopped coming. Earl's treatment didn't work either, and he had pretty bad cirrhosis. He became our gentle, steady voice for the perils of delay, influencing countless new patients in ways that he probably never appreciated. Then Earl developed liver cancer. He couldn't get a liver transplant and he eventually died. That was hard on everyone, and we still miss him.

Through all these ups and downs, new members would become involved and invite friends, family, and what might be called "associates" to join us. All were welcome, as long as they behaved. Tim Maginnis is another one of my wonderful peer educators, but he was quite the sight when he started showing up at our program. "Tore up from the floor up" is how he describes it. Remember that character Pig-Pen from the comic strip *Peanuts*, who always had a cloud of dirt around him? Well, that was Tim but the cloud was alcohol. He would drink a fifth of vodka just to get up the gumption to show up—not to mention the heroin, cocaine, and whatever else he was using at the time. But he was always polite, and he always listened. He stopped drinking alcohol and smoking crack, began taking methadone to stop using heroin, and eventually got off the methadone. In the process, he became one of the most insightful and knowledgeable patients I have ever had. But the booze and hepatitis C had done their thing: His liver biopsy showed cirrhosis. So we treated him and then he was cured. But even after that, he kept showing up. I eventually got tired of that and hired him.

There were a lot more stories like this, and the group kept growing. We eventually started a second group on a different day. And at some point we came to regard the groups differently.

They had begun as a strategy to help our patients, but we instead came to see ourselves as the primary beneficiaries. Our first treatment challenges were minor compared with those that we faced later: more complex layers of drug use, mental illness, and instability that represented the real face of hepatitis C, not the one we were hoping for. We had kept our belief: You don't have to die of hepatitis C. Our group was the tool we needed.

We no longer concerned ourselves with who might or might not be stable enough for treatment. We found that was hard to predict, so we just let our patients prove themselves. Show us that you can show up each week, every week. Prove it, and we will offer you treatment.

That was an unusual concept. Most of us have fixed ideas about good or bad treatment candidates. The majority of hepatitis C patients in my practice would probably have been considered bad candidates or worse. There was often some element of instability to factor in, such as drug use, mental illness, or homelessness. These are the things that most doctors avoid. But what is it about these things that keeps us from treating hepatitis C?

Mostly it comes down to adherence. We question their ability to follow instructions and take medications. We question their willingness to attend follow-up visits. We question their commitment to complete therapy. These are all reasonable concerns, because they could affect safety as well as outcomes. But we are especially questioning of patients who are not like us.

And so when a patient shows up at our clinic, we often end up with a lengthy list of problems to address. Sometimes hepatitis C can be high on the list, but not always. If it is, if hepatitis C treatment is a priority, then we consider it our ethical duty to figure out how to offer it in a timely fashion.

Many doctors have a strategy with hepatitis C: I won't

help you with it until you do these other things. Those are the rules, I am the doctor, you do what I say. Come back in six months. Chances are, with the kind of patients I see, they won't ever come back. Maybe that is part of the strategy.

But I don't like people dying of hepatitis C when effective treatment is available. And I am not the boss of anyone, never having been appointed. So here is the deal: You come to our groups. We will treat you like family. You will learn everything you care to know and more about hepatitis C, testing, and treatment. In the process we can make sure that we are both committed to the same goals. And when those things have happened, I know you'll be safe, and treatment can start.

With that unconventional approach, the benefits grew. Patients would show up inebriated, intoxicated, resistant to care. In addressing their hepatitis C, they became motivated to stop drinking, stop using, build new bridges to health, reconnect with family, return to work. Not necessarily in any particular order, but who am I to decide what is right? As their doctor I take what I get.

All this has got me thinking about transformative experiences and hepatitis C. The idea of a transformative experience is an interesting one. You are one person, then you have some experience or other, and because of it you become someone else.

So I started asking people what they would consider their transformative experiences. People I know outside the clinic, more mainstream people, would almost invariably come up with something like having their first child, or getting married, or perhaps taking a particular job. Things that amounted to mundane, scripted, and societal occurrences.

But when I asked that same question of some of my patients, people who'd also been married, had kids, and had jobs, I got very different answers. "Mainlining smack the first time." "My first bump of coke." "The first time I got loaded." That sort of thing.

The difference is, these really were transformative experiences: A key was inserted, the tumbler turned. Unlucky genetics collided with adventurous stupidity. One event, and from that moment on an endless cycle of getting drugs, using drugs, withdrawing from drugs, poverty, violence, homelessness, and incarceration. Failure, from society's standpoint. Perhaps some drug treatment, but usually not much to speak of, unless you put incarceration in that category. Where will that kind of money come from? Employer-based tax credits?

Most of my patients were kids at the time. One of them has been hooked on heroin since she was nine years old. Think about yourself at that age, and consider it.

At some point there is an aftermath: hepatitis C, its acquisition never once a transformative event, having gone unnoticed in the chaos. Then time passes and they show up at our clinic. But as you have seen, hepatitis C is not our end, it is our means. For us, it is our carrot, a way to attract patients with far more pressing and challenging problems. We use hepatitis C to convince our patients that who they really are is not who they seem to be at the time. They are not bad people. They are good people with a very bad problem.

I have never thought of that as a transformative experience. But I suppose it is.

Chapter 8

Advocacy

Chris comes to advocacy honestly; it is in his blood. I myself am a latecomer. It was not part of my training. It's not what we doctors do. This mess of our health care system is a consequence of that.

In a small way, though, I have seen its benefits firsthand. On a number of occasions, we have taken our patients to the State Capitol to educate our legislators about hepatitis C. Many times, legislators visibly startle when patients identify themselves as addicts. I am proud that my patients are willing to do this. It tells me that we have taught them well, that they understand addiction is not a shameful condition but instead a medical condition that responds to treatment. The surprise of that disclosure changes the tone of the meeting in many good ways.

My patients have brought our hepatitis C educational materials to the Sacramento office of every single state assemblyperson and every single state senator, and they have business cards to prove it. They brought me one extra card last time we were there, and it was from Gov. Arnold Schwarzenegger's office. As you will see, it appears that we are getting somewhere here in California, hard as it is to accept the glacial pace.

If you have hepatitis C or know someone with it, by all means that should be your priority. But many others could use your help. It may not seem as if you make a difference by getting involved, but you do. I hope you will consider doing so.

I had no idea of the level of infection in this country, in the world. Even though I'd gone through treatment, I knew nothing about the bigger picture of this illness. So I learned and part of what I learned is that nobody knows enough. On the most basic level, we don't even really know the scale of the HCV problem we're facing, because there's no budget and no plan for surveillance. Just to explain: In public health terms, surveillance doesn't mean wiretapping or anything like that. It's an organized, systematic way of gathering information on how many cases of a disease are diagnosed and treated within a given population. There are some state programs for HCV surveillance—and I'll talk about them in a minute—but there's really nothing in place nationally. The Centers for Disease Control has the authority to do this kind of work, but they have no money. The CDC's Division of Viral Hepatitis (which covers both hepatitis B and C) has a budget of about seventeen million dollars a year. That money has to cover not only the division itself but also outreach efforts in the fifty states and six U.S. territories. It pays the salary for one adult viral hepatitis coordinator in each location, but that's about it. So there's no federal testing or treatment programs, which means we have no good national data on hepatitis C. The information we do have is pretty dire. We think that there are almost three million Americans infected with HCV, but the number could be as high as six million. You want to know the scariest thing? About 50 percent of people currently living with hepatitis C have no idea they're infected.

Because there's no national leadership on HCV, treatment is dealt with mainly on a state level. In a time of tightening budgets, states often squeeze funds for HCV testing and treatment from existing HIV programs. It's a great idea to build on the successes of structures already in place, instead of reinventing the wheel. And it makes a certain amount of sense to combine treatment and outreach for the two diseases: Rates of coinfection are significant, and there's overlap in the at-risk populations. But when the budget has to stretch to cover two programs, neither one is adequately funded and they both suffer. You would think it would be simple for the HIV folks, who are very well funded, to shave off a little bit of money for HCV, and that that little bit would go a long way. But it doesn't happen, because when you have a billion dollars, you spend a billion dollars because you've created a system of care that needs a billion dollars.

When I first became aware of the prevalence of HCV I didn't understand how an illness that affects four times as many people as HIV could be left with so few resources. The fight against HIV is well funded because the diseases are different, and that affects the way the public responds.

HCV doesn't kill people as quickly as HIV did in the early days, before effective drug cocktails. And hepatitis C isn't nearly as easy to transmit. With HIV it was clear that if it wasn't addressed aggressively it could sweep through the whole population. That's not the case with HCV. The people who were on the front lines of the AIDS epidemic were organized, well funded, and focused. That's not happening with hepatitis C, for lots of reasons. For one thing, half the folks who have it don't know they have it. For another, the current new infections are primarily among drug-addicted and prison populations, where advocacy is virtually nonexistent. This also means that people outside those populations don't feel threatened by hepatitis C.

But this lack of serious advocacy for HCV, coupled with the lack of broad, coherent standards and policies, can risk serious outbreaks. In February 2008, six cases of HCV were traced to a clinic in Las Vegas, Nevada. An investigation by the Centers for Disease Control found that health care professionals at the clinic had been reusing syringes and medication vials, as well as cutting corners on sanitary measures. The unsafe practices had been going on for as long as four years and put more than forty thousand people at risk. By May 2008 eighty-five cases of hepatitis C had been linked to the original facility and an associated clinic. With national prevention policies in place, the outbreak might have been avoided—or at least detected earlier.

There are efforts under way to get the necessary policy changes through Congress. In May 2007 I was proud to watch my uncle Sen. Edward M. Kennedy introduce the

Hepatitis C Epidemic Control and Prevention Act, which would begin to address some of the problems. The bill directs the Secretary of Health and Human Services to develop and implement a nationwide plan for the prevention, control, and management of HCV. It would finally establish nationwide standards for best practices in preventing spread of the disease, integrate hepatitis C testing into the existing public health infrastructure, and educate the general public and health care workers in order to increase the number of people diagnosed. This bill has been introduced with bipartisan support for each of the past three congresses but has yet to make it into committee.

After he introduced the bill my uncle met with me and two patient advocates, Michael Ninburg, executive director of the Hepatitis Education Project, and Lorren Sandt, the hep C program director at Caring Ambassadors. Uncle Ted explained the political reality we're facing, on a couple of different levels. For one thing, there's Sen. Tom Coburn of Oklahoma. He's a physician, a radical-right Republican, and a member of the Senate Committee on Health, Education, Labor, and Pensions. He's also totally opposed to any disease-specific bills—like the Hepatitis C Epidemic Control and Prevention Act—and he works to block them from ever getting out of committee.

That's just one individual's personal agenda, and it might be easier to overcome his opposition if we were talking about a different disease. In Washington and in the state capitals, it's tough getting politicians to pay attention to hepatitis C. Currently the disease is primarily associated with populations that have no political capital: current and former drug addicts, and those who are incarcerated. These people are not organized and often don't—or can't—vote, so politicians generally don't pay much attention to them.

So those of us who are trying to change things point out that the majority of Americans infected with HCV have never used drugs or been in prison. We tell those who will listen that this is a disease that adversely impacts our veterans and first responders, and that hep C can be sexually transmitted or passed between the mother and child during pregnancy or birth. And we use the numbers. We tell legislators that there are at least four times as many people with hepatitis C as people with HIV. Most people who are coinfected with both HIV and HCV will die of HCV-related complications. Each year, somewhere between eight and ten thousand Americans die from HCV and related complications. That annual death rate is expected to keep going up, reaching as high as twenty thousand by 2030. That's *deaths*. That doesn't include everything that happens on the way—like liver transplants at upward of $300,000 a pop, for an uncomplicated case. Like end-stage liver disease, including cirrhosis and liver cancer, which can cost anywhere from $31,000 to $110,000 per hospital admission. We're talking about billions of dollars in medical costs, dealing with the long-range effects of HCV. Now compare that with the cost of actually treating hep C. Depending on the protocol, total treatment costs range from $15,000 to $25,000, with a 55 percent cure rate, and there are new drugs in the pipeline that promise a 10 to 20 percent increase in treatment efficacy. The numbers are clear, and the fiscal conservatives get it. At least, some of them do.

I've talked with legislators in Pennsylvania, Georgia, Florida, and California. In Atlanta, I met with Rep. Earl Ehrhardt. I didn't get very far—not because he didn't care or was unaware of the problem. Though he's a conservative Republican, Representative Ehrhardt has hosted the state's Hepatitis C Day for three years running. As a member of the House Appropriations Committee and chair of the Rules Committee, he's very plugged into the workings of the state legislature. He told me, "Chris, I've got ten boxes full of data from around the state of Georgia on this disease. You're asking me for funding, and I don't even have the money in the state budget to hire someone to open those boxes and go through them."

We had better results in Pennsylvania. I met with Republican state representative George T. Kenney Jr., chair of the Health and Human Services Committee. That guy gets it. Working with Joanne Grossi, deputy secretary of the state Department of Health, Kenney actually shook loose $250,000 for surveillance in Pennsylvania to see how big a problem they're facing. This was the first time a state actually funded HCV testing and education. Combined with a matching amount of federal funds, they started five HCV testing sites in Pennsylvania. As part of this program, methadone clinics were supplied with kits for testing people in high-risk populations. In the first three years of the program they've tested over seven thousand people in Pennsylvania. More recently there's been discussion of the need for programs focusing on HCV case management, to encourage people identified through testing to actively pursue and complete HCV treatment. Unfortunately state funding for existing and new programs is up in the air. Kenney retired at the end of 2008 and Grossi has moved to another position. We've got to keep the pressure on.

There are some very good state programs around the country, ones that most researchers and advocates consider useful, workable, and flexible models that can be replicated anywhere to begin addressing the hepatitis epidemic. The programs in Florida, Illinois, Iowa, New Mexico, and Texas are considered especially successful and innovative. I've included some details on those programs, and links for more information, at the back of the book. If you live in one of these states, consider getting acquainted and getting involved with these people. The good news here is that there's important work going on to fight hep C at the state level. The bad news is that all this progress is endangered by budget cuts and shortfalls—a problem that is only going to get worse.

One thing I've noticed over the years is that the states with the best HCV policies tend to be the states with strong, well-organized advocacy groups. That's definitely true of California. CalHEP was formed in 2006 to address the wide disparities in HCV treatment throughout the state. From the beginning the group has included both people affected by HCV and medical professionals who specialize in treating the disease, and I think that range of expertise and experience is one of the keys to its success.

Early on we made a decision to focus on policy efforts to combat hepatitis B as well as hep C, and we've made some progress despite California's ongoing budget crisis. Currently CalHEP includes fifty member groups, with advocates targeting local issues throughout the state. I have had the privilege of serving as honorary chair for CalHEP through a very busy 2008.

In March we headed to Sacramento for the first Hepatitis Advocacy Day, where state policy makers were educated about the scope and consequences of viral hepatitis in California. That was where I met Diana Sylvestre and we had our first conversations about doing this book. We also managed a meeting with Governor Schwarzenegger to plead our case for funding. Though he was sympathetic, he wanted to know who was going to pay for it because there was no money in the state budget.

In the 2008 California legislature, Assemblyman Mervyn Dymally (D–Los Angeles), introduced legislation to require the California Department of Public Health (CDPH) to develop a program for the prevention of liver cancer and liver disease caused by viral hepatitis. CalHEP sponsored this legislation and shepherded it through the Health Committee, where it passed 8 to 4, and into Appropriations, where the bill died as a consequence of California's budget crisis. I know from my uncle's experience in Washington that it can take years to pass significant legislation—persistence and coalition building are key— so we'll be back as often as it takes, and each time we will bring more allies.

• • •

Here's the most important sentence in this book: *Hepatitis C has a cure.* There was a time when medical professionals didn't like to talk about curing this disease, but that time is past. Those of us who are fighting HCV can use the word *cure* now, and we should. In the next few years, the cure rates for genotype 1, the most common one, will top 60 percent. Genotype 2, the one I had, already has a cure rate of 75 percent. When I was in denial and delaying treatment, it took a while for that fact—the fact that I could be cured—to sink in. When I finally got it, that's what motivated me to start treatment. That treatment both saved and changed my life.

If I had not been tested, or if I'd remained unwilling to be treated, I'd be dead now, or close to it. I'd be dealing with transplantation, liver cancer, or end-stage liver failure. That was the road I was headed down, and yet I have a life today, my kids have a father today, and I am contributing to our society today because I was tested, diagnosed, and treated. And I was lucky. Two of the things most precious to me—my sobriety and my cure—came to me because I was lucky. I didn't do anything to deserve them; I just finally had sense enough to grab them and hold on to them when they came to me. There are at least four million Americans who should get the same chance I had. Not because they deserve it, but because it's the right thing to do, and because it makes sense.

I believe addiction and hepatitis C are no-fault diseases and that the possibility of recovery from these illnesses should be an opportunity given to anyone who wants it. As individuals and as a society we have an obligation to advocate for surveillance, prevention, and treatment for all of our citizens, regardless of where they may fall in the social or economic order. We can look at this in economic terms: The money spent on treatment and prevention saves us money in the long run. Or we can look at it as a question of simple human dignity and respect, of keeping what we have by giving it away. Either way it's the right thing to do.

For the first thirty years of my life I was a taker, and for the last twenty-three I have tried to give back. There are millions of others out there just like me who, if given a chance, will turn their lives around and benefit our society instead of depleting it. In recovery I have many friends who have done just that, only to come face-to-face with the life-threatening disease of hepatitis C. That's why I can't walk away. That's why I am committed to being a voice speaking out against the stigma and discrimination rampant in the way addiction and hepatitis C are viewed. A voice demanding that our society treat these illnesses the same way it treats other chronic, life-threatening diseases. A voice asking all of us to stay focused on the underlying societal causes and conditions that lock people into hopelessness and despair.

After a lifetime of trying to be what I thought everyone wanted me to be, I've found my true self in everything I was ashamed of and tried to hide. I am somebody today not because I make movies and give speeches and write bestsellers but because I give back. I get to use my experience, strength, and hope to help others change their lives. I'm not doing this because I'm a good guy. I'm doing it because my own life depends on it.

And if you're at risk for HCV, your life depends on three things: Get tested. Get treated. And get cured.

That bears repeating: Get tested. Get treated. And get cured. Or as we say in my clinic, you don't have to die of hepatitis C. Look, I realize we're not quite there yet but we're getting close. In my short time doing this, treatment response rates have gone from 15 percent to 40 percent to 55 percent, and the next bump upward is headed our way soon. There is hope for everyone to beat this disease and even to eliminate it from the planet, but not unless we choose individually and as a society to make that happen.

Now let's get right down to what this book is really about: Is there actually a cure for hepatitis C? Here's a message from the countless thousands of supposedly unreachable people we have educated at the O.A.S.I.S. clinic, from the more than 3,500 rejected patients whom we have screened, and from the many hundreds of untreatable hepatitis C patients whom we have successfully treated. And from Chris and me, from all of us: We'll take the odds. Yes. Yes, there is a cure for hepatitis C. And you can quote us on that.

Online Resources

While these are all useful sources of information, they're no substitute for talking to a health care professional who knows you and the details of your condition. Educate yourself, get support from your peers—but always consult with your doctor before taking action.

Information Clearinghouses

O.A.S.I.S. (Organization to Achieve Solutions in Substance-Abuse)
http://www.oasiscliniconline.org/
This is Diana's amazing clinic, which provides low-cost, subsidized medical care to medically marginalized former or current drug and alcohol users. They've developed some great books and videos explaining hepatitis C and its treatment—and it's all free.

Hepatitis C University
http://www.hcvu.org/index.php
O.A.S.I.S shares their hard-won expertise in treating hepatitis C through this educational Web site designed for health care providers. Using this site, treatment providers receive expert mentoring through the innovative HCV Fellows Program offered free of charge.

HCV Advocate
http://www.hcvadvocate.org

An excellent site, including a function to find local HCV support groups. Their "Living with Hepatitis C" page has lots of practical advice for understanding and dealing with insurance claims and disability filing.

http://www.hcvadvocate.org/hepatitis/living_w_hepatitis_C.asp

To contact them or to request materials by mail: alanfranciscus@hcvadvocate.org

Hepatitis A, B, and C Prevention Programs
http://www.hepprograms.org/index.asp

This Web site showcases programs across the United States that work to prevent hepatitis A, B, or C in people who are at risk for infection. Links to prevention programs, support groups, and related topics, including needle safety.

Caring Ambassadors Hepatitis C Program
http://www.hepcchallenge.org

This national nonprofit organization is devoted exclusively to meeting the needs of the hepatitis C community, offering state-of-the-art information and awareness building. Their "Disease Management" page has a wealth of information, including a map of HCV testing sites throughout the country: http://www.hepcchallenge.org/disease_management.htm

HIV and Hepatitis
http://www.hivandhepatitis.com/

A comprehensive gathering of news reports and information on FDA-approved and experimental treatments for hepatitis C, as well as hepatitis B and HIV. Especially useful for those who are coinfected.

Online Support Group

HCV Support http://hcvsupport.org/forum/index.php

If you can't find a local HCV support group, or if you just want a place to vent at 2:00 a.m., this is a good resource.

Insurance Issues

Patient Advocate Foundation http://www.patientadvocate.org/index.php

This national nonprofit organization "seeks to safeguard patients through effective mediation assuring access to care, maintenance of employment and preservation of their financial stability relative to their diagnosis of life-threatening or debilitating diseases." Not HCV-specific but very useful.

HMO Help http://hmohelp.ca.gov/default.aspx

Obviously this is going to be most helpful for California residents, but it's very good at explaining HMO terminology and structure, which are pretty much the same throughout the country.

Centers for Medicare & Medicaid Services, Medicaid Ombudsman
http://www.cms.hhs.gov/center/ombudsman.asp

This is a good overview on federally funded Medicaid: who's eligible, how to apply, where to go for help.

Enrolling in Clinical Trials

Clinical Trials http://clinicaltrials.gov/

Easy-to-navigate site explaining how to find and apply to be included in clinical trials. When I searched for studies on "Digestive System Diseases," I found more than two hundred HCV studies that were looking for participants.

Workplace Issues

Social Security Disability
The Benefit Eligibility Screening Tool (BEST)
http://connections.govbenefits.gov/ssa_en.portal

This online questionnaire helps you figure out if it's worth applying for temporary benefits. It's not an application, and it doesn't link to your personal Social Security number or records in any way.

Disability Insurance
U.S. Department of Labor Employee Benefits Security Administration
http://www.dol.gov/ebsa/publications/filingbenefitsclaim.html

A general guide to filing for benefits offered through a company or individual policy.

United Policyholders Tips on Disability Insurance Claims
http://www.unitedpolicyholders.org/claimtips/tip_disability.html

United Policyholders was founded in 1991 as a non-profit tax-exempt organization dedicated to educating the public on insurance issues and consumer rights. They mostly focus on disaster insurance and claims, but this page has many useful tips and links on disability insurance.

Family and Medical Leave Act

U.S. Department of Labor Family and Medical Leave Act Advisor
http://www.dol.gov/elaws/esa/fmla/faq.asp

The FMLA, passed in 1993, guarantees eligible employees at any company up to twelve weeks of unpaid sick leave. This page gives you a rundown on who's eligible and how FMLA protection works.

State Efforts

Because so much of the fight against HCV takes place at the state level, we wanted to draw attention to some of the best programs we've come across. Some of these are ongoing, while others have been cut short by ever-present budget problems. But all of them show how talented, dedicated professionals can come up with creative, innovative solutions. Where it's available we've included contact information for these departments or services.

Florida

In 1999, the Florida legislature appropriated $2.5 million to the Florida Hepatitis and Liver Failure Prevention and Control Program, which covers hepatitis A and B as well as HCV. The legislature also authorized approximately $3.1 million per year in subsequent years for hepatitis prevention and control. These programs for testing and outreach are administered by the Bureau of HIV/AIDS of the Division of Disease Control of Florida Department of Health (FLDOH) and works collaboratively with the HIV Prevention section. From 2000 through 2003 the Florida program administered more than 34,000 doses of hepatitis A vaccine and more than 65,000 doses of hepatitis B vaccine. During the same time period approximately 67,000 pieces of educational material were distributed, and two radio spots promoted HCV testing.

Florida Hepatitis Prevention Program

http://www.doh.state.fl.us/disease_ctrl/aids/hep/index.html
Information on free testing in Florida: 850-245-4334

Illinois

In 1999 the Illinois Department of Public Health (IDPH) established successful pilot programs to test and treat viral hepatitis at selected STD/HIV clinics. Though they had to scramble for funding, the pilots were successful enough to expand it statewide the following year. Also in 2000 a CDC Viral Hepatitis Integration Project (VHIP) grant enabled IDPH to pilot six health department sites to provide targeted HCV testing to IDUs at six sites, selected based on population risk data, STD morbidity, and ability to integrate comprehensive viral hepatitis prevention services into HIV and STD prevention services.

Although funding for VHIP ended and hasn't been replaced, the project produced an enormously useful database of information about viral hepatitis spread and treatment, allowing them to improve clinic efficiency and effectiveness.

Iowa

The Iowa Department of Public Health provides HCV counseling and testing through integration with STDs, substance abuse, and HIV prevention programs. The state uses HIV prevention funds to pay for HCV testing for high-risk clients in these programs. The CDC-funded HCV Coordinator manages the HCV integration programs. The state's three-day counseling and testing training for HIV program staff includes comprehensive modules on STDs and HCV. Organizations applying for HIV program funds must offer HCV education and testing services. Participating programs receive a small amount of funding for staff and are required to use the state laboratory for testing.

In May 2006 the legislature passed the Iowa Viral Hepatitis Program and Study, which will be supported with tobacco settlement funds. A small amount of funds were appropriated to support HAV/HBV vaccination and HCV testing of populations at risk. Hepatitis and HIV/AIDS advocates joined together in Iowa to form Community HIV/Hepatitis Advocates of Iowa Network (CHAIN). Together these advocates work to educate state policy makers about the need for increased prevention and care funding for both HIV and hepatitis. They don't take a one-disease approach but advocate for the needs of all Iowans impacted by either HIV or hepatitis.

New Mexico

In New Mexico state general funds support comprehensive HCV prevention, education, and treatment services, as well as an adult hepatitis A and B vaccine program. These services are fully integrated with HIV prevention and education programs. The New Mexico Hepatitis C Alliance was born in 2003 from a consensus conference sponsored by the New Mexico Department of Health, the University of New Mexico, and conference members and stakeholders. The alliance developed the New Mexico Hepatitis C Strategic Plan and has put the plan into action. One very cool element of the plan is Project Echo, funded by the state and operated by the University of New Mexico. Through the wonders of video and broadband Internet, Project Echo allows people in prisons and remote rural communities to get access to HCV treatment.

New Mexico Hepatitis C Alliance
http://www.nmhepcalliance.org/

NMHCA
P.O. Box 1106
Albuquerque, NM 87048–1106
Phone: 505-314-6555

Project Echo
http://echo.unm.edu/

Yolanda Hubbard, Community Education Coordinator
1001 Medical Arts Ave NE, Bldg 424
Albuquerque, New Mexico 87102
yhubbard@salud.unm.edu
Phone: 505-272-9875
Fax: 505-272-6906

Texas

Texas has been pretty cutting edge in dealing with HCV. The Education and Prevention Program for Hepatitis C was established in 1999, and required the Texas Department of State Health Services to offer specialized training to health care professionals, set up outreach efforts, and figure out the impact of HCV on the state's residents. Since then the funding has dwindled to less than a tenth of its original levels, but the initial push helped set up workable infrastructure integrated into existing HIV programs. Despite the chronic lack of money, they've managed to maintain their counseling services and ongoing training, offered to both HIV counselors and licensed chemical dependence counselors. The sites that don't offer HCV testing themselves are able to refer clients to low-cost testing through the state health department.

Texas Department of State Health Services
An overview page on their Hepatitis C initiative
http://www.dshs.state.tx.us/idcu/disease/hepatitis/hepatitis_c/overview/

California

As we described in the advocacy chapter, one of the ways to affect state policy is through a strong advocacy organization. The one we know best is CalHEP. In 2008 we didn't get our bill through the legislature, but we did establish an alliance with the California Department of Public Health (CDPH), in which we committed to developing a strategic plan to address viral hepatitis in California. At a September 2008 planning meeting, CDPH and CalHEP agreed on the following priorities:

Driving policy change. For example, needle exchange is only available on a county-by-county basis. CalHEP advocates for lifting the national ban on federal funding to support needle exchange and for California to implement needle exchange as a statewide program.

Educating the public and providers about viral hepatitis. This would include a culturally competent public awareness campaign targeted to communities disproportionately affected by hepatitis. There are way too few providers trained to treat hepatitis, especially in community health clinics where the vast majority of patients are seen.

Targeting and integrating hepatitis services into appropriate programs. We want to build on the existing infrastructure that reaches people at higher risk—drug and alcohol treatment programs, needle exchange programs, HIV testing and treatment settings, and STD clinics.

Improving the surveillance system. Right now there's not a system in place to identify people who are diagnosed with chronic hepatitis. Without good data we'll never be able to address hepatitis successfully and target our approaches where they are most needed and most effective.

California Hepatitis Alliance
1330 21 Street, Suite 100
Sacramento, California 95811
http://www.calhep.org/
Phone: 916-930-9200
Fax: 916-930-9010

Acknowledgments

To my doctors and their nurses for getting me tested, diagnosed, and treated, saving me from the horror of liver transplantation, cancer, or death.

To my uncle Senator Edward Kennedy for his example and tireless commitment to bettering our health care system.

To the hep C advocates across the country who dedicate their time and energy to raising awareness about this disease, especially Lorren Sandt of the Caring Ambassadors Program, Michael Ninburg of the Hepatitis Education Project, and Pam Langford with HEALS of the South.

To Martha Saly of the California Hepatitis Alliance and the National Viral Hepatitis Roundtable for her invaluable research assistance.

To my good friends Bill Kennedy, Kale Browne, and Andrea Davis, who—with great patience and no judgment—listened to me rant and rave ad nauseam throughout my treatment.

To Loretta Barrett for her hard work making this book happen, and her ability to forgive.

Finally, to my kids, who endured my treatment, and to

Jodi and Taylor, who endured the writing of this book—I love you all.

—*Christopher Kennedy Lawford*

To the O.A.S.I.S. Clinic medical staff for whom decency and justice were reason enough: Amy Smith, PA-C; Barry Clements, PA-C; Jane Garner, PA-C; Laphyne Barrett, MA; Rosa Sanchez, MA; Lisa Molinaro, RN, MSN; and Deborah Greene, MD. Your work has changed the face of hepatitis C.

To our peerless peer educators Larry Galindo, Tim Maginnis, and Gerard Wallace, whose thoughtful advocacy has grown more hope and saved more lives than you ever could imagine.

To those mentors whose wisdom and insights helped smooth my rough edges and kept me from coloring too far outside the lines, especially Joan Zweben, PhD; Judy Martin, MD; and Mary Jeanne Kreek, MD.

To Brian Edlin, MD, and Karen Seal, MD, MPH, whose research expertise helped spawn our program.

To Christopher McNeil, secretary from hell but eventually videographer extraordinaire, who helped put our education strategies on the map.

To Bridget Branch and Andy Hansen, whose calm, kind, and deliberate demeanors help forestay clinic pandemonium.

To Jan Werner, for creating order out of chaos, and without whom this book would not exist. You really should be with us on the front cover.

To Charles, my first and only love. Why you put up with me, I will never know.

Acknowledgments

And especially to the countless O.A.S.I.S. peer volunteers who have given tirelessly of themselves. You have inspired me with your strength, your hope, and your dedication. Without you, our program would be nothing at all.

—*Diana Sylvestre, MD*

Index

Index